10-12.71

HEALING AND WHOLENESS

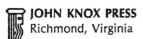

HEALING and WHOLENESS

Edited by D. WAYNE MONTGOMERY
with an introduction by
HOWARD J. CLINEBELL, JR.

JOHN KNOX PRESS
Richmond, Virginia

Grateful acknowledgment is made to the editor of *The Journal of the American Medical Association* for permission to reprint selected articles from the years 1965–1969. The article "Medicine and Religion" first appeared in the August, 1965 issue of the *Denver Medical Bulletin* and was reprinted in the December, 1965 issue of the *Rocky Mountain Medical Journal*. Reprinted with permission in this volume, *Healing and Wholeness.*

International Standard Book Number: 0–8042–1115–9
Library of Congress Catalog Number: 77–152888
© John Knox Press 1971
Printed in the United States of America

1621657

ACKNOWLEDGMENTS

Gratitude is expressed to John H. Talbott, M.D., editor of *JAMA,* not only for permission to reprint the articles but for encouragement to do so, also, the Reverend Paul B. McCleave, Director of the Department of Medicine and Religion of the American Medical Association, and Mr. Arne Larson, Assistant Director, for their guidance and assistance in tracing down the contributors, mainly, I think, through the efficiency of Mr. Larson's secretary, Reneda A. Mittman!

Howard J. Clinebell, Jr., Professor of Pastoral Counseling, School of Theology, Claremont, has given a focal point for all of the articles in his Introduction. I am expressly appreciative of this gesture as the beginning of my doctoral work included two courses from him, who at the time was visiting professor at The Iliff School of Theology.

The manuscript and all that was necessary for its preparation was made possible by Dr. Paul W. Renich, President, Kansas Wesleyan. Joan Foss, department student secretary, did all the detail work plus typing the manuscript, with the exception of bringing together the loose ends, which fell to my office student secretaries Nancy Willcox and Roann Perryman.

I wish a proper gesture toward all the contributors could be that of listing their publications—but a reading of them is startling—and humbling. So, this mention will have to suffice.

TABLE OF CONTENTS

PREFACE

This book is about medicine and religion—not as disciplines separate unto themselves, but as interrelated approaches to the treatment of the patient and the family. The total health of man is contingent upon his well-being: physically, spiritually, emotionally, and socially. Of necessity, then, the healing process must be multi-faceted, with the physician and clergyman being those two professions upon which the mantle has fallen.

The Department of Medicine and Religion of the American Medical Association announced that its sole purpose "is to create the proper climate for communication between the physician and the clergyman that will lead to the most effective care and treatment of the patient." With the exception of the Introduction, the paper on "Medicine and Religion," and Conclusion, the following articles are from the pages of *JAMA (The Journal of the American Medical Association)*. All have something to say about the totality of man, his worth, and his value as a person, together with guidelines concerning a cooperative ministry in the treatment of the whole man.

Within these pages are many opportunities for creative dialogue among members of the two disciplines, and allied professions. A careful reading of the material reveals that the concern for the care and treatment of the patient and his family has never been more total than now. The future is even brighter!

The introduction into a cooperative effort on the part of the physician and clergyman first came into my life in a pastorate where the five physicians of the community were all a vital part of my ministry. To them I owe much concerning the value of human life—especially one with whom I stood on many occasions. I am very appreciative of those men in St. Francis, Kansas, who considered all of us in a ministry together.

JAMA was introduced to me in the home of James H. Gentry, M.D., Denver. Of particular interest at the time was the magnificent art work on the covers, and the advertisements which provided preaching material. Dr. Gentry, as well as physician friends in other locations, saved his copies for my use.

Areas of primary concern are treated in this collection of articles, but with the growing ecological crisis others will need treatment also. Perhaps someone reading this collection will muster the time and resources to do so.

These articles do not purport to be definitive answers to the problems explored. This is a cross section of what representative doctors, clergymen, and others are thinking as they cope with the problems of the patient, knowing that most often his needs far transcend the physical ailments for which he seeks help.

The contributions are interfaith and interdisciplinary: priests, ministers, and rabbis; physicians, professors of medicine, psychiatrists, and psychologists; medicine, religion, and law; Catholic, Protestant, and Jew—all are represented, but with a common purpose—the treatment of the whole man.

These resources are commended to you. May they expand your horizons and enlarge your perspectives of the meaning of man and the role you are to assume in his treatment. May it assist in bridging a gap which need not exist.

Fall, 1971

D. Wayne Montgomery
Kansas Wesleyan

INTRODUCTION

Howard J. Clinebell, Jr.

The *need, opportunity,* and *resources* for clergy-doctor collaboration are greater today than at any previous period of
history. In a society that fragments persons and relationships, it
is imperative that the healers get together. Otherwise, they will
continue to contribute to the splintering of contemporary man. It
is particularly important that the healers of the body and clergymen, the healers of relationships (with self, others, and God),
learn to work together more effectively as they deal with the
same individuals and the same families. Around such an axis of
cooperation, it is possible and desirable that other healers—
social workers and clinical psychologists, for example—may join
in new professional alliances dedicated to releasing trapped
human potentialities.

In some ways, clergymen and physicians are natural allies.
These two professions share certain strategic opportunities with
respect to helping and healing: both are present during many of
the crisis periods when mental/physical/spiritual health hangs
in the balance. Both have reasonably regular contacts with the
majority of the culture's personality molders—parents. Family
physicians and parish ministers, in contrast to most other professionals, have a direct entrée to the majority of family con-
stellations, *the* crucial social organisms in the society. Clergymen
and nonpsychiatric physicians do the great bulk of counseling on
personal and family problems in this country (71 percent in one
well-known study: 42 percent by clergymen and 29 percent by
doctors). The kinds of counseling which are most effective, for

use by parish ministers and the nonpsychiatric physicians, are very similar. Both professions are interested in the "whole man," yet neither has the training that equips it to respond to all the needs of the whole man. The training and skills of each profession complement those of the other. This key point is spelled out with clarity in several of the papers in this book.

New opportunities and resources for clergy-doctor collaboration and cooperation have been created by developments in recent years. The clinical teaching of pastoral care in seminaries has begun to pay off in producing a growing group of clergymen who have learned under supervision the skills of interprofessional dialogue and cooperation. The presence of well-trained chaplains and pastoral counselors on the staffs of an increasing number of agencies and institutions has helped to educate medical and paramedical professionals regarding the valuable role of the clinically sophisticated clergyman on the healing team. The community mental health movement has created new settings for and a new impetus to interprofessional teamwork, as mental health leaders have recognized the tremendous untapped mental health potential of our country's 300,000 plus clergymen. The presence of a clergyman with theological and psychosocial training on the staffs of community mental health services has proved to be a vital factor in achieving the community goals of those services, goals which require widespread interprofessional collaboration. Certainly, the growing interest among nonpsychiatric physicians in psychosomatic medicine provides a natural link between their concerns and the central concerns of clergymen for spiritual and societal health. Some recent trends in theology support the shared interests of ministers and religiously oriented physicians in the spiritual dimension of wholeness.

Candor requires one to recognize that our record of interprofessional relations in the past, has been nothing to shout about, except perhaps in protest. With some notable exceptions, distancing between clergymen and physicians has been painfully prevalent. The territorialism, mutual ignoring, stereotyping, and one-upmanship which have occurred among all the "helping" professions have frequently vitiated fully effective helping of the burdened, troubled, or sick person. We've talked a lot about teamwork, but actually practiced it much too infrequently. The time obviously is ripe for a breakthrough in the achievement of what one paper in this volume describes as "a firm, cordial working relationship" among the various helping professions, including doctors and clergymen.

Several things are essential if greater teamwork is to flourish. Of central importance is mutual understanding and appreciation of each other's unique competencies, views, insights, and contributions to the helping-healing enterprise. Each needs a robust sense of professional self-esteem, which is affirmed in interprofessional relationships. The willingness and the opportunity to communicate are also crucial, as is the openness to learn from each other. (Interprofessional communication has frequently been comparable to making love through a picket fence—a somewhat distant and very strained transaction.) Another essential of increased doctor-clergy teamwork is more frequent opportunities to work together in helping the same patient/parishioners. Maximum mutual learning results from such experiences when there is in-depth dialogue and reflection on what happened in the actual encounters with each other and with the persons being helped.

This book is a useful resource in the achievement of several of the essentials just enumerated. Its major contribution is in making some of the medical literature which is relevant to the interests of clergymen accessible to them. (To keep the flow of the learning process two-directional, there is a need for a companion volume of papers by clergymen to be read by physicians.) Readers will be impressed by the insights and spirit of outreach of the doctors who write on the need for clergy-doctor teamwork. Less than a third of the papers deal with interprofessional cooperation, per se. The great majority discuss areas of joint concern —e.g., the sexual revolution, telling the terminal patient the truth, the issue of prolonging life vs. prolonging dying, the ethical questions raised by organ transplants, and other advances of modern medicine. Focusing on such areas of overlapping interest would seem to be a greater stimulus to interprofessional cooperation than a heavy concentration of the process and problems of this cooperation.

The paper entitled "Medicine and Religion" states well the goal of interprofessional dialogue and collaboration: "The heart of the matter . . . lies in individuals of each profession coming to know, respect, and understand their opposite members so that they may meet at the bedside as colleagues and consultants." This book is one resource for developing such colleague-consultant relationships. The editor has done the fields of pastoral care a service in selecting these papers and drawing them together under one cover. The book complements the previously available literature in the field of doctor-clergy interaction. It makes a significant contribution to that interaction and therefore should be a factor in the much-needed emergence of a new era of interprofessional collaboration.

MEDICINE AND RELIGION

William Carl Bailey, M.D.
and Bernard T. Daniels, M.D.

In 1961 the AMA Board of Trustees created a committee on Medicine and Religion composed primarily of physicians, but also of several nationally prominent clergymen of various faiths. This committee was charged with the responsibility of bringing the forces of medicine and religion together, based on the premise that "whole man" is a physical, mental, emotional, and spiritual being, and that to effectively care for him the understanding, knowledge, and skills of all branches of medicine and religion must be brought together. To meet this responsibility the Committee recommended and received financial support for a strong administrative arm, the Department of Medicine and Religion.

Component Societies—Heart of Program

In this new venture, a great deal of effort was expended by the Department in gathering information, organizing pilot programs, and attempting to determine needs. One of the most important first tasks has been the establishment of organizational machinery for the program's development. State society committees on Medicine and Religion have now been formed in each state. These committees have, in turn, assisted county or component societies to organize their own committees. The latter local groups constitute the real heart of the program, for it is here that direct contact between practicing physicians and clergy must be made.

The organizational structure of the program, therefore, follows already existing lines. This natural outgrowth has advantages: in avoiding duplication of organizational effort, and in facilitating the ready exchange of information, ideas, and evaluation of results through long-established and effective routes of communication.

Medicine—The Common Denominator

Direction of the program at national and local levels is under medical rather than primarily religious leadership for several reasons. Certain broad generalizations may be made about the significance of religion in the lives of patients, whether atheist, agnostic, or devout believer. The great diversity, however, of faiths and shades of religious belief among individual patients (and doctors) presents a bewildering contrast to the relatively uniformly accepted body of scientific knowledge and medical practice. Therefore, in this interdisciplinary effort, medicine appears to be the common denominator. Medical leadership has the advantage that it can cross lines of religious conviction without the encumbrance of particular denominational thrust.

While the doctor must continue his primary role as the provider of medical care in the historic tradition, the major purpose of this program is to bring doctors to accept that portion of responsibility for the patient's spiritual needs which is also their legitimate concern. This can best be done by doctors themselves within a medical framework.

Interest in Importance of Religion

With the goals of the program in mind, it is worthwhile to examine the means by which it is hoped to achieve them and some of the problems being confronted. One of the first and most easily predicted difficulties has been that of the selection of committee personnel. The uncharted areas into which the program must move made substantial demands on committeemen, requiring hard work, imagination, straight thinking, and charity. To be effective, the committee member need not profess any particular religious faith, but he must have a lively interest in the importance of religion (and of nonreligion) in health and disease. He must have adequate time to devote to the committee, personal conviction, and yet be capable of necessary clinical detachment.

Developing committees composed of physicians who meet these requirements has taken time and effort. It has, on occasion, been tempting to consider partially staffing committees with members of the clergy. Carefully selected clergymen with a clear understanding of the purpose of the program have, in fact, on occasion, lent great strength and increased effectiveness when brought into such committees. However, a nonsectarian atmosphere must be maintained if the program is to be effective; it is understandably more difficult for the clergyman to divest himself of his denominational point of view than for his medical counterpart to do so. Too great reliance on the clergy has, therefore, to be avoided.

Role of Laymen

The question has been properly put: why have an organizational program when the matter is really an individual one? The answer is not difficult. It is quite true that the best committee is a committee of two—one doctor and one clergyman, working together for one patient. But unless . . . the two professions can meet as a group and discuss their mutual problems more frankly than in the past, there is scant likelihood of improving the relationship between one doctor and one clergyman over that which now exists. The need appears to be for dialogue between physicians and clergy, not only as individuals, but as organized groups.

It is easy to talk enthusiastically about the need of a program such as this. Interest in the "whole man" has been rekindled by studies in psychology and psychosomatic medicine. There has been a renewal of religious interest in all spheres of activity, in and out of science and the professions. This has been particularly evident in Europe. On all sides there is talk of ecumenicity, new appreciations of the common origins of Judeo-Christian theology, and a keener and more sophisticated interest in those religions which are not so familiar to us in America. The role of

the dedicated layman has recently achieved new respect and
recognition, and there are few occupations which so readily lend
themselves to the lay ministry as does medicine. Within the
areas of medicine, psychology, and the social sciences, there is
growing awareness of the importance of religion even among
professionals who may themselves be nonreligious. Among
theologians very exciting things are happening. Basic theological
concepts are being reevaluated and profound efforts are being
made to bring religion to direct confrontation with the problems
of space-age society.

Problems of Physicians and Clergy

All of these factors make it easy to obtain acceptance of the
concept that "something should be done" to promote cooperation between medicine and religion for the benefit of the sick in
a manner and degree never previously considered.

But obviously little will be accomplished if the discussion
collapses in a morass of high-sounding, but empty, oratory, and
thought does not produce the fruit of purposeful activity. Our
purpose must be to bring the concept to the patient at the most
effectual human level.

The average physician knows extraordinarily little about the
place that religion truly occupies in the life of his individual
patient. The same may often be said of the minister or rabbi.
Tactful and skillful "history taking" and the knowledge of how
that patient's religious "set" affects his pathology (and the converse) frequently are the marks that distinguish the amateur
from the professional in either profession. The clergy is often
appalled by the callous, if innocent, indifference exhibited by
the doctor toward his patient's spiritual needs, let alone the lack
of a working knowledge of the basic tenets of that patient's
specific religion. On the other hand, how many physicians have
been indescribably annoyed by inept religious ministry, by a
lack of medical sophistication on the part of the clergy which
may exceed that of the patient, and even possibly by conduct
which he may find questionable by standards of medical ethics?
These general statements barely serve to indicate the number

and depth of the problems which face physicians and clergy in their joint efforts to provide better care for sick people.

The purpose of the Department of Medicine and Religion is to stimulate dialogue which, it is hoped, will meet and help solve some of these problems. At a practical level the organization of programs which will do this has met difficulties. Physicians and clergy face enormous demands on their time in the form of various organizational meetings, not to mention those made on them in the actual practice of their professions. There are considerations also in arranging meetings of the two professions for formal or informal discussion. The size of the community may have a bearing. The smaller rural communities of a dozen or less physicians and a comparable number of clergy have found it easy to meet and to discuss problems of the community, individual patients in whom there is common interest or concern, as well as to enlighten each other about specific medical and theological applications. The heart of the matter, of course, lies in individuals of each profession coming to know, respect, and understand their opposite members so that they may meet at the bedside as colleagues and consultants.

Establishing a Friendly Relationship

The mutual education of large segments of each profession and the establishing of comfortable and friendly working relationships between doctors and clergy presents vastly more complex problems in large urban areas. In these communities the chances are slight that the physician and clergyman mutually involved with a given patient will even be acquainted, let alone have a firm, cordial working relationship with each other. In this connection, although their role is not yet fully developed, the professional hospital chaplains have helped fill a great need. By virtue of special training they are often remarkably conversant with medical practice, have a sophisticated appreciation of the intricacies of the interrelationship of disease and religious belief, and in many cases have developed a clinical point of view which, far from rendering them a sterile influence, makes it possible for them to minister to many of the sick in situations where a more parochial approach would be highly ineffectual. They are usually well known to the staff physicians, and by their credentials and on the strength of past performance are frequently welcome consultants. But, the assumption that such highly skilled professionals can fulfill the entire need of either the patient or the program of the Department of Medicine and Religion, is invalid. However skillful, the hospital chaplain cannot take the place of the personal religious leader, even aside from denominational or faith differences. In addition, there are relatively few such chaplains available and, even if their number were adequate, the need to better educate the leaders of the religious community about the effects of illness continues to be a serious one. Hospital patients go on to become not only outpatients in doctors' offices, but members of congregations.

In the education process, considerable thought has been given to the type of program vehicle which will be most interesting and fruitful. Formats vary with the size of the community and the resources available. It appears that a useful size working group can often best be attained through the utilization of the subcommittee comprised of the hospital staff, which brings clergy and doctors together in a pattern of common interest, geographically and professionally. Every effort must be made to use all of the talent and other resources available in the community in informed discussions, lectures, seminars, and workshops. A highly effective discussion technic, widely used, and applicable to a group of any size, is that of the clinico-pathological conference. This is an excellent, proven technique with which physicians and clergy are comfortable, and which lends itself beautifully to the discipline of reducing theory to practical application.

Recognition of Mutual Concern

Whatever the circumstances, the size of the community, the talent available, or the organizational machinery, the sole aim of the Department of Medicine and Religion is to improve patient care. The concept of the wholeness of man far antedates modern medicine, as any student of medical history is fully aware. This renewed interest in the unique interrelationship of physical and spiritual health is, in fact, nothing more than a manifestation of acceptance by modern physicians of a basic characteristic of the human creature. The "new" element is that it is being emphasized and developed by organized medicine. The results of the program will exceed our expectations if the momentum of its inception can be continued by its medical leadership, if it can be kept patient-centered, and if it can maintain the historical values of medicine and avoid the quagmire of denominational dispute.

The spiritual health of every man profoundly affects his physical and mental well-being. Physicians and clergymen have much to gain for their patients and parishioners and nothing to lose by recognizing their mutual concerns and working together.

THE PATIENT AS A "WHOLE MAN"

There has been a great deal of recent publicity in the lay press and in scientific periodicals about the changing patterns of the practice of medicine. The medical profession has been accused of being "impersonal" and it is a current fad to denounce the physician for "not taking a more personal interest in the patient." Many of these criticisms emanate from biased sources, of course, and not infrequently the critic is unaware of the fundamental changes in diagnosis and therapy. I would appreciate comments from your consultants in the form of a candid discussion of what the physician's concept of his professional obligations to his patients should be. Have the salutary effects of medical progress been accompanied by an unfortunate erosion of the personal identity of the patient? What do we mean by the consideration of the patient as a whole man?

RESPONDENT: *Melvin A. Casberg, M.D.*

Within the past few decades medical knowledge has increased at a rate undreamed of by physicians of the recent past generations. Scientific information doubled in the first half of this century and has doubled again in the past ten years.

In such an environment of explosive growth and change, the physician of necessity focuses on an ever narrowing field of activity, fragmenting the patient into organ systems and even their lesser components. Diagnostic and therapeutic gadgetry presents an expanding maze of technical equipment extending the healing arm of the physician. Morbidity and mortality statistics continue to react favorably and dramatically to the rapidly advancing vanguard of medical discoveries. Yet there is an uneasiness in the minds of many physicians that this very progress poses a threat to the personal identity of the patient and his treatment as a whole man.

No serious thinking person would revert to the days of the horse and buggy doctor, with his well-intentioned but woefully inadequate means of practice, and yet, this dignified citizen of the community of yesterday, respected and loved as a physician and counselor, dispensed medicine with a compassionate understanding so essential to the healing of the whole person. Unfortunately, in this age of scientific efficiency, far too often the impersonal mechanics of modern medicine have crowded compassion to a serious degree.

The same scientific pressures which are forging new tools for the diagnostic and therapeutic armamentarium of the physician are creating tensions in a modern society increasingly besieged by fears and uncertainty. In such an environment, breeding loneliness and insecurity, where the dignity and personal identity of man may suffer from the very magnitude of the scientific revolution, it becomes critically urgent that we physicians nurture a mutual concern for the whole man. Unless we can approach the patient in the delicate terms of human values, our profession will lose the warmth of mutual respect and the strength of moral stature, each so essential to balanced medical therapy, and evolve into a science of cold materialism dealing in the problems of health and disease with the detachment of the scientist who conjugates amino acids.

Man is a unique composite of an inscrutable triad fused into a single being which Holy Writ informs us was created in the image of God. The perceptive physician must be aware of these separate but interrelated facets of the body, the mind, and the spirit, and appreciate that healing the body in the face of a broken mind or spirit is but a partial victory, or even an ultimate defeat. In the face of this mystical nature of man the scientist must realize that the material master key alone cannot unlock the storehouse of health.

We speak of a balanced endocrine system or a coordinated muscular action in glowing terms of physical well-being; however, in considering the whole man, the symmetrical maturation of the body, the mind, and the spirit is essential in the broadest concept of health. As pitiable as is the housing of a sound mind in a broken body, how much more tragic and dangerous is the asymmetry of a deformed spirit unequally yoked to a superior intellect.

Ingenious apparatus and techniques for the assessment of the physical status of the patient are available to most physicians, but no such equipment exists for the determination of this same individual's level of spiritual well-being. This latter subjective facet of man does not lend itself to evaluation by the standard objective qualitative or quantitative tests of science. And yet, how critically significant is the intimate personal spiritual faith of the patient. How deeply this affects the health of the whole man.

It is not the physician's place to don the cloth of the clergy and function in an area of theological or spiritual concern without proper qualifications, but it is his responsibility to recognize that man is a person with a spiritual birthright whose substance is far greater than the mere sum of his material components. The concept of a team approach, namely, the physician and the priest, in the care of man's illness, is as ancient as the history of man himself. With all due respect for the accepted functions of the man of the cloth, the physician with a personal religious faith can play a significant role in the strengthening and stabilizing of his patient's spiritual well-being.

Some eight centuries ago, the Persian poet Saadi, with a remarkable insight in the relationship of the physical and spiritual components of the whole man, wrote: "Should'st thou repair, then, to thy larder and there, find of all thy once bounteous store, but two loaves remain, I yet counsel thee to sell one wherewith to buy white hyacinths to feed thy soul."

THE PHYSICIAN'S OBLIGATION
TO HIS PATIENTS

Every physician has a uniquely personal concept of his professional and personal obligations to the person he serves. These views are inevitably influenced by the particular role in medical practice for which he has been trained. A clinician in general practice and two physicians engaged in a specialty practice were asked to give their personal views concerning obligations that go beyond mere professional competence and which are peculiar to the discipline of medicine they have chosen. Following are statements by a general practitioner (Dr. Peeke), a plastic surgeon (Dr. Monroe), and an obstetrician and gynecologist (Dr. Hulit).

RESPONDENT: *Alonzo P. Peeke, M.D.*

The general practitioner has an advantage over the specialist in his close and intimate association with the patient and his family. A good general practitioner can take care of 85 percent of the medical needs of a person. The specialist, by limiting his practice to a single organ system and to certain limited types of procedure, has fewer opportunities to see patients in a variety of desperate and commonplace situations.

The general practitioner becomes an integral part of the family from the time of the birth of the child. His services are sought for vaccinations, communicable diseases, accidents, and behavior problems. If father gets ill the wife tells him to go to her doctor, and so the whole family becomes the concern of the general practitioner. He becomes interested in each member of the family as an individual in every phase of the family life, the education of the children, their successes after graduation, as they settle in other parts of the country and the world. He is intimately associated with civic and church interests, which provide a common bond of association with the patient. The doctor even takes an interest in the love affairs of the children growing up, the marriages, and all the important affairs of the family— including the final illness of some of the family members. His association with the community and the knowledge of his patients' church affiliation makes it easy for him to contact their pastor or priest.

The day I received the request to prepare this communication, I had an experience which illustrates the general practitioner's role. Most farm accidents occur after 5 p.m. This may be due to hurry or fatigue or a combination of both. An excited man called me to come quickly to a farm seven miles southwest of town where a silo was being filled. He said there had been a bad accident. The corn was being cut and blown into large covered wagons, each of which has a space of two and one-half feet from the front into which the silage is deposited. There are rollers with spikelike revolving projections which move the silage back into the wagon. The machinery is driven by a power take off from the large tractor. A wooden roller block had broken and become wedged in the chain which drives the rollers. The operator had dismounted from the tractor without shutting off the power take off or tractor, and had crawled up into this two and one-half-foot space to see what was obstructing the normal operation. His clothing became impaled on the rollers as he was trying to move them, and he was pulled into the rollers and killed. He was alone. About ten minutes later, his employer found him.

Here was a thirty-six-year-old man whom I had delivered as a baby and known all his life, a fine, hard-working farmer with a wife and eight children under ten years of age. You can imagine the sudden impact of all the things which had to be done immediately: the ambulance to be called, the pastor to be notified, and then the task of visiting the widow to break the news to her. Supper was ready and waiting, the children had done their chores and were waiting for their father to come home. The pastor got there just before I came. There was not much we could do for the father, but just think of the immediate things which had to be done. Think of the future things to be done for the young, growing family. We have for years been stressing farm safety in 4-H organizations, extension work, and the Rural Health Program of the American Medical Association. This was another urgent impulse to speak and participate in farm safety programs, which is prophylactic medicine.

I submit that the place of the general practitioner in rural America is involvement in every phase of the family life and in all phases of the community life. The family physician cannot say, "This is not in my field and I am not qualified to do this," or "I have put in my eight hours," or "Why should this family's religious, emotional, or economic life involve me, a doctor?" We have so many more opportunities to be called on for help because we treat the whole man and have not limited our usefulness. We cannot disregard the spiritual or social or economic life of our patients.

RESPONDENT: *Clarence W. Monroe, M.D.*

The patient who seeks out, or is sent to, a plastic surgeon is primarily concerned with having competent work done. This may range from making a small scar less obvious to straightening a slightly crooked nose, to reconstructing half a face removed for cancer or rebuilding a thumb lost in an accident. Would that it were always possible to achieve each of these objectives with complete perfection! The patients would surely be happier, but it is doubtful whether the simple technical skill to achieve such routinely happy results would long remain a challenge to the men who have sought training in plastic surgery.

The patient with a problem which can be only partially corrected constitutes the technical challenge of plastic surgery.

But it must also be recognized that each patient who seeks our help has another problem concerning his own body image. Even the person who has a small scar and seeks to have it made less obvious or completely obliterated has, by the very act of seeking the plastic surgeon, admitted a mental concern for a perhaps insignificant deformity. The surgeon may see the immediate possibility of accomplishing the patient's wish in toto. He may, therefore, agree to the proposed procedure without further ado. However, he is often wiser to take a few minutes to find out why such an insignificant deformity concerns the patient enough that he is willing to go through an operation. The answers to gently probing questions may reveal other facets of the patient's character which make it unwise to do the operation.

Contrariwise, the first interview with the parents of a newborn infant with a cleft lip and palate must offer them a great deal more than the simple promise of a well-repaired lip. Such parents are usually revulsed by the appearance of their own child and are overwhelmed by a mixture of repugnance and pity. They would prefer either to shun the infant completely or smother him with tender loving care. It is the surgeon's duty to take them verbally through the steps of repair with a realistic appraisal of the child's chances for good appearance, good teeth, good hearing, and good speech. And he must expect that they will hear only a fraction of what he tells them on the first visit. But it must be said, and said again and again, until the child is reared as any other normal child.

In such a child, as in many other types of deformity or injury, it may not be possible to repair the patient so well that *no* stigma is left. However, the plastic surgeon must feel that he has failed, in part, in his care of the patient if he has been unable to persuade the patient to live with reasonable equanimity with that portion of the deformity which cannot be corrected. This sometimes proves a more difficult task than the surgical repair. Yet to stop short of treating the whole patient in this manner is to fail in our management.

The reward for this approach to the patient's problem is his everlasting gratitude in most instances. When the patient is convinced that the surgeon has done his very best in a technical and esthetic sense, and at the same time has been honest and forthright in admitting that the end result falls short of the perfection that patient and surgeon were seeking, the great majority find themselves able to face the world unafraid.

RESPONDENT: *Bob E. Hulit, M.D.*

Consideration of a doctor's obligations beyond mere professional competence brings to mind an anonymous saying, "Life is like a game of tennis; the player who serves well seldom loses." Concern and kindness and service are not scientific requisites for the practice of medicine, but they certainly are desirable attributes in the specialty of obstetrics and gynecology.

Concern for the pregnant woman's role as a wife and as a mother to other children is basic to good prenatal care. Kindness that relieves unreasonable fear or frustrating tensions is essential for the best management of labor. Taking the time to explain and having the patience to listen are necessary criteria for superior gynecological therapy. A kind of competent practice of the specialty is possible without these extras, but the mother delivered of a baby she rejects is not much improved. The tranquilized grandmother, who is still lonely and convinced she is no longer needed, has not been treated at all.

Specialization of any type is not a license to treat a segment of a person. In obstetrics and gynecology, the diseases treated are peculiar to women, but the care of a female child involves her parents; treatment of a wife relates also to the husband; and responsibility for a mother embraces the entire household. The parents, the husband, and the family are all a part of the patient. Some diseases can be treated and cured apart from this total patient, but there are many instances when concern for her must be inclusive of all such segments of her total health.

I wish I could describe myself as one who always treats the total patient, and fulfills all of the responsibilities over and above required competence. My examples are shadows of my conscience more than actual case histories. Under the pressures of time and patient load and self-interest, I compromise between what is required and what could be done, between what is right and what is good.

I think first of the unmarried teenage mother-to-be, so frightened by her disaster that adequate examination is barely possible and so convinced that her world is near an end that she scarcely knows where she is. The doctor's best treatment might be limited to confirming the diagnosis she already knows and covering up his personal prejudices about unmarried girls based on moral standards he accepted many years ago. This might indeed "do no harm"! The obligation beyond mere competence, however, includes accepting the patient as the person she is, planning for her prenatal care and delivery, and assuring her of support and help which will eventually include cooperation with parents, social worker, and clergy. This is the help the girl requests by coming to the doctor's office, and this is the treatment she should expect.

Premarital examinations are done by members of the obstetrics-gynecology fraternity with more variation in content and quality than any other specific phase of the specialty. The different ideas of responsibility to the patient are mixed with all sorts of variables in interest, moral judgment, time allowed, rapport, and follow-up. Competent treatment is something more than making a serological study and retailing a Baedeker to conjugal bliss. A competent and adequate physical examination is a must. With the New Morality, it takes great insight and perception to be sure of the patient's motivation. A contraceptive method is desired by most patients, whether they are really anticipating the first sexual encounter or have already had sexual experience. Basic sex education is seldom what the patient is seeking, but for those few who need it, the omission could be a tragedy. Some evaluation of the patient's concept of sexuality, with relevant insights and advice, can be a real contribution, regardless of the patient's basic motivation. The type of modesty or fear that keeps a wife and a mother from going to a doctor when something is obviously wrong seems incomprehensible and inexcusable in this day and age. Just as a child needs to be loved most when he is most unlovable, the patient who has deliberately ignored her abnormal bleeding or the lump in her breast until it seems hopeless needs consideration beyond mere specialized competence. She is aware of her mistake and wishes now that she had come sooner. What her neglect may mean for her children and her husband is already on her mind. The tragedy of her regret and sense of guilt is further compounded by an irrepressible human "Why me?" remorse.

The very best treatment given with superior competence is too often a delay of the inevitable. The physician with a conscience feels frustrated by medicine's inadequacy and wonders if the fear or false modesty may have been iatrogenic in any way. Responsibility beyond competence becomes a whole series of moral decisions: in allaying the patient's guilt and remorse; in helping her to accept her disease; in solving the enigma of the patient protecting the family and the family protecting the patient; and in involving clergy and agencies in the treatment. The ministry of kindness becomes part of competent treatment and may be what will do the most ultimate good.

Further instances when required competence may not be adequate treatment are numerous: the weary-mother syndrome; fertilities studies; the menopause patient; the geriatric woman. The patients come with complaints that are just a hint of the real problem. The symptom named is a key, and it takes real courage to go ahead and open Pandora's box. But hope was also in Pandora's box, and the patient has been given only symptomatic relief until the total problem is recognized.

There is tremendous satisfaction in being a part of the scientific achievements in medicine today, but keeping abreast of the new knowledge added to any single specialty is a formidable and required responsibility. Further subspecialties may become necessary before cybernetics provides the promised answers. Computerized medicine will make many doctors more efficient and scientifically competent, but in obstetrics and gynecology a very special type of programmer will be mandatory if the type of patient and problem I have described still exists. If the programmer does not have the concern and kindness to go beyond the stated symptoms, the real problem will never get into the machine, and what comes out will be chaos.

PHYSICIANS, CLERGYMEN, AND
THE HOSPITALIZED PATIENT

I am a medical administrator in a hospital which includes medical, surgical, and psychiatric departments. Patients with a variety of diagnoses, ranging from peptic ulcers to schizophrenia and anxiety neuroses, are treated here. The clergymen who visit patients of their respective religious groups have often expressed a certain inadequacy in regard to their background in technical psychiatric training. What are the respective roles of the psychiatrist and the clergymen in the care of the patients? Can a minister offer constructive assistance to a patient who is under psychiatric care?

RESPONDENT: *Gotthard Booth, M.D.*

Throughout the course of history most physicians have recognized that in all forms of illness the morale of the patient influences the effectiveness of therapeutic procedures. Sir William Osler, one of the greatest teachers of medicine, stressed: "It is more important to know what sort of a patient has a disease than what sort of disease a patient has." The old-fashioned physician, even in the beginning of this century, had very few physical means of controlling disease processes, but he had great opportunities for restoring and supporting the psychological health of his patients. He was usually personally known to them as a man trusted by his family and his community. The physician from his side could usually gain easily knowledge of the character of the sick and of the psychologically significant circumstances of his life. The custom of house-calls, in particular, conveyed quickly and without words many facts which are difficult to discover by verbal exploration in office or hospital. All this provided the doctor with a basis for strengthening the spirits of his patients because he could address himself to concrete factors in the human situation.

The modern American physician finds himself caught in a dilemma which he cannot escape or resolve singly or with the help of his medical colleagues alone. On the one hand, psychosomatic research has provided more and more scientific observations which demonstrate the influence of psychological conditions on functional and organic diseases; on the other hand, he has less and less time for establishing psychological contact with his patients, because the progress of physical and chemical research is making more and more strictly physical procedures necessary. For the conscientious scientific doctor, his patient is becoming increasingly a bundle of laboratory figures which reduce his awareness of the suffering human being. The more serious the illness, the less opportunity there is for any personal encounter between doctor and patient.

The minister has a unique opportunity for helping in the situation which medical science has created. He can and should keep his mind free from all the details connected with the disease proper so that he can concentrate fully on the person on whom he is calling. Often he is in the position of the old family doctor as far as the establishment of personal rapport is concerned. If the patient comes from his own parish he knows more or less the individual history and family background. Even the hospital chaplain has often a certain advantage over the physician in case the patient happens to be a total stranger. A common religious background provides a basis for communication whereas, due to the heterogeneous and mobile character of the American population, physician and patient are liable to have a very few personally significant experiences in common. The sharing of values provides a basis for the *humanitarian* function of the minister. The function is, first of all, to rescue the patient from the self-absorption into which everybody tends to sink as the result of the disease itself, and of its practical consequences. The most important of the latter is hospitalization which is the concomitant of all serious illness and separates the sick patient radically from his normal psychological environment. Even before the advent of hospitals, visiting the sick (Matt. 25:36) was recognized as a crucial responsibility because the experience of illness not only causes disruption of human relationships, but often it is also evident that illness has been a consequence of some loss and grief.

The patient is apt to receive a minimum of relief from the mere experience that the minister is visiting him, even if his religious affiliation should be of a rather nominal character. Obviously those with deeper religious feelings will be helped by prayers and sacraments. Although it is not within the province of the medical man to discuss pastoral procedure, some points may be made regarding the role of the minister as a person. Now that the medical profession has become widely concerned with ministers as important participants in its therapeutic work, many ministers feel burdened with a much greater sense of their own responsibility. At the same time they are faced with the awe-inspiring machinery of powerful medical methods which tend to make them feel weak and their words too immaterial to be of any account. Particularly in the presence of threatening or inevitable tragedy the insecure ministers are tempted to match the depersonalized medical procedures with a depersonalized religious approach. The offer of a prayer, if made by a minister trying to hide his own anxiety, is not very helpful to a severely frightened patient.

In addition to becoming a huge technological apparatus, medicine has developed in still another direction which has made many ministers insecure in their pastoral approach: I am referring to psychoanalysis. Its scientific discoveries about the complexities of the unconscious mind and the consequent improvements of psychiatric therapy have created the unfortunate prejudice that ministers should either get psychoanalytical training or confine themselves to a bland, nondirective bedside manner which is supposed to be nevertheless "supportive." Some ministers have been so impressed by warnings of how easily unconscious anxieties might be aroused that they are even afraid of offering prayers and sacraments. These conclusions about psychoanalysis are unrealistic and confusing for the minister who wants to be a minister and not a psychotherapist. Obviously the latter vocation calls for psychoanalytical training regardless of the academic background. Most hospital cases, however, are not in need of depth therapy, and even many inmates of psychiatric institutions can benefit from pastoral care. As a matter of fact, the clinical training of ministers originated in a psychiatric hospital forty years ago thanks to the initiative of Chaplain Boisen.

Boisen concluded from his own experience as a former inmate of a state hospital that the most important need of the sick is "to be restored to the human fellowship" from which their illness has separated them. For this purpose he concentrated the clinical training of ministers on the development of an individualized relationship with the patient. Nothing is more depressing for the latter than to feel reduced to the status of being "a case of . . . ," even if this should be sugarcoated with the administration of T.L.C. On the other hand, nothing is more supportive than to feel recognized as a unique person who is suffering from some type of more or less common ailment. The latter experience is conveyed by the minister who makes himself acquainted with the specific concrete realities of the patient's life. Instead of questions about the patient's feelings and more or less convincing reassurances about medical prognosis, questions should be aimed at his life situation before the illness began, how it affects his relationship to family and work, and what he expects regarding his future existence. This procedure is more effective and not necessarily more time-consuming than a nondirective exchange of platitudes. It provides obviously also opportunity for pastoral comment. Even psychotics often retain enough contact with reality to communicate with a minister who is not afraid of down-to-earth facts. For psychotic patients this approach is actually even more important than for normal individuals because psychotics are quick in sensing insecurity behind generalities. The average medical and surgical patient is approachable by a minister who takes genuine interest in the conscious problems of the people. Certainly organically sick individuals also have an unconscious mind and unconscious conflicts. This realm, however, should worry the minister as little as cholesterol levels, X-ray films, etc. Occasionally a patient may behave in a peculiar way which calls for a psychiatric opinion, but this is likely to happen as frequently as the need to call the medical doctor or surgeon on account of some acute physical symptom during the visit.

If the minister tries to modernize his function by striving to become also a psychotherapist, he foregoes the unique advantage which his calling gives him in working side by side with the physician. As pointed out in the beginning, the healing of a disease depends on two equally important conditions: the medical treatment of the sick condition of the body, and the morale of the person. Because the minister does not need to occupy himself with what is sick, he is free to strengthen what is healthy. By relating himself to the patient as one human being to another, he brings the sick in closer contact with his religious resources. The more serious the disease, the greater is the help which the minister can give by reducing the fear of death, one of the greatest dangers to recovery. Last, but not least, if recovery should be impossible, the minister can reduce terminal pain and anxiety.

RESPONDENT: *Abraham N. Franzblau, M.D.*

There is no question that ministers and physicians can not only coexist amicably today, but can cooperate in many fruitful ways. There are, of course, tender areas between them which have to be handled with care, and even areas of possible conflict which have to be resolved.

Today not hundreds but thousands of ministers have had clinical training in hospitals and correctional and other institutions. This has brought tremendous awareness of the pastoral role and contribution to the clergy itself, but even more important, to the medical profession. On the other hand, members of the clergy are being appointed to the faculties of medical schools, many psychiatric associations have standing committees on psychiatry and religion, and there is a growing amount of literature in the field. All this constitutes a happy ferment.

However, if maximum benefit is to accrue from the cooperation of physicians and clergy, it is important to clarify the role of the minister in pastoral counseling which, properly practiced, is a distinct and separate entity from psychotherapy.

The minister is uniquely situated for his pastoral duties. He has the opportunity, week after week, to communicate with his flock from the pulpit, the religious school, and the vestry. In their homes, he enjoys a unique privilege available to no other professional, that of unannounced calling. When a couple wish to marry, they must meet whatever standards and requirements he sets up, and he is party to occasions of joy and sorrow in their lives. They turn to him for marital counseling, for help in child-rearing crises, and for guidance in many other problems. Despite the uniqueness of his role in his parish, some of these problems border on the realm of the psychiatrist, and this is where some conflict may arise if sharp and clear boundaries are not set up.

The minister has a wide range of permissible activities, many of which are wholly forbidden to the psychiatrist. He can offer advice; the psychiatrist cannot. The relationships of the minister are meant to be enduring, sometimes going on to the second and third generation. The psychiatrist's are intentionally self-limiting; the more effective he is, the less needed he becomes as the patient grows in inner strength.

The minister may also correct and castigate his parishioner. The psychiatrist cannot. People expect their minister to "speak out" against every form of immoral or unethical conduct, whether in the private or public domain. In some confessions the minister has the privilege of according or withholding absolution for sins, a position foreign to the role of the psychiatrist.

In tragedy, the minister can afford consolation and solace, and offer helpful services and goods to the individual or the family. This is wholly outside the function of the psychiatrist. Even in the depressions accompanying bereavement, the minister is there on the spot and is usually able to help more than the psychiatrist.

The minister speaks not only for himself, but for his church. As a listening ear, he is invested with his charisma, standing as the representative of God before the parishioner, according him recognition and worth; hence, the individual may walk away greatly helped by this fact alone. The minister belongs to all of his people, all of the time, while the psychiatrist belongs to a very few patients, and only for a few fixed hours. The minister can teach and inspire, strive to renew courage and increase strength, clear clouded vision, and restore judgment. The psychiatrist may not do any of these directly. The minister, believing in the efficacy of prayer, can add this to his other contributions. When, however, does the minister reach the border line which limits the boundaries of his proper function as a pastoral counselor? When should he call in a psychiatrist?

When the minister deals with a parishioner's problems, he deals with them in a context of normality, as minor disfunctions, and can therefore operate with impunity as a pastoral counselor. When the problem grows more serious, involving a breakdown in the person's capacity to function normally in his family relations, his work, his social relations, his ethical values and behavior, or his ideational processes, then the minister, even if he is trained in pastoral counseling, is wise to make a referral to the psychiatrist, who is trained to handle abnormal mental and emotional conditions and ailments.

Psychotherapy is something very different from pastoral counseling. It is a branch of the medical practice of psychiatry, based on a specific dynamic psychological theory and utilizing a carefully controlled scientific technique. It requires a broad background of medical knowledge and skills, as well as years of special psychiatric training and experience. The best that the well-trained psychiatrist has to offer is sometimes inadequate. For ministers to meddle in psychotherapy without the same training as psychiatrists have is unjustifiable. It is not enough to have a few months of clinical pastoral training, a few courses in psychology, some "supervision," and some personal psychoanalysis. There should be no back doors into this realm.

If a minister is determined to enter the practice of psychotherapy, he really should study medicine and undertake training in psychiatry. However, with a Ph.D. in psychology and good basic training in psychotherapy, he could function as a psychotherapist in an institutional setting under the supervision of a psychiatrist. However, this is in most cases tantamount to leaving the ministry and entering the paramedical field. Very few of those who have followed this course in the past are still in the ministry today.

The growing border of the relationship between our two professions, medicine and religion, must be carefully safeguarded, if a healthy structure is to result.

DISCLOSURE OF MEDICAL INFORMATION TO CLERGYMEN

Does a member of the clergy have the right to obtain medical information from a physician without the oral or written consent of the patient involved?

Does a member of the clergy have access to medical records in the hospital without oral or written consent from the patient? Is it necessary to have permission from the attending physician also?

Does a member of the clergy have the privilege to obtain information concerning a medical or psychiatric consultation if the patient specifically requests that the findings be absolutely confidential between patient and physician?

RESPONDENT: *Richard P. Bergen, J.D.*

A physician or hospital may properly disclose medical information about a patient without the patient's consent when such disclosure is required by law or is necessary to protect the best interest of the patient or to protect the public. In some circumstances disclosure of information to a member of the clergy might be justified on this basis.

Apart from these exceptions, no disclosure of confidential medical information should be made without the patient's consent. The physician's consent is not necessary for disclosure of hospital records, if the patient consents.

Unless disclosure of information to a member of the clergy is necessary to protect the best interests of the patient, the member of the clergy has no greater right to this information than does anyone else.

PHYSICIANS, CLERGYMEN, AND
THE PRIVILEGED COMMUNICATION

The minister in our church is also a close personal friend. He has on a number of occasions suggested that I, as a physician, should be aware of the fact that there are some discrepancies in the current attitudes of physicians toward communication with clergymen. It is his opinion that he has frequently been unable to be of maximum service to his parishioners because of the medical profession's lack of understanding of the role of the clergymen in counseling and supporting the ill. What is your frank opinion of the intent as well as the implementation of the concept of privileged communication between physicians and physician and clergyman? Do you believe that physicians are inclined to assume functions which more properly belong in the realm of the ministry?

RESPONDENT: *Rev. William J. Fogleman*

The physician ought to be always first and foremost concerned with what happens to his patient, and therefore honesty or integrity in any legalistic sense is a commodity which the physician cannot afford!

The physician is always in a position to reveal or withhold whatever facts or insights he may have and should do so only on the basis of his judgment of how such revelations or withholdings affect the health of the patient. By health is meant the total well-being of the patient. Physicians in their professional roles are always under obligation to remain the means to an end, for this is what it means to be a "professional." It is not possible to make a hard and fast rule, therefore, concerning honesty and communication. The law of Christian love and demands for health and well-being on the part of the patient forever may legitimately override the virtue of honesty. It is the context of the situation which determines the degree to which the maxim "Honesty is the best policy" should be honored.

Honesty in communication with the clergyman by the physician should also be in the context of a particular situation. A physician must make some assessment of the ability of the clergyman to use intelligently, creatively, and benevolently whatever communications he shares. Under the best of circumstances, complete honesty and reliance on the professional integrity of physician and clergyman would be the pattern. In this respect, the physician needs to discover that frequently the clergyman, because of his long and continuing relationship with the patient and the family of the patient, has much to contribute to the physician's understanding of the current situation of illness at hand.

The whole matter of privileged communication between physicians needs serious rethinking. This clergyman discovers time and time again that where physicians are eager to maintain the status of privileged communication between doctor and patient, they will frequently share with another physician (who is in no way involved in the case in point) casual observations or reports on the patient or his family or both. Another physician who is in no way involved with the case in hand should have no more access to privileged communication than any other layman is privileged to have.

The whole area of philosophical questions, it seems, has particular bearing on the nature of the training available in medical school and the kind of continuing education physicians receive. Physicians, because of the particular roles they perform, are continually being thrust into life situations for which they have little training and on which they seem not at all inclined to reflect. While they object to clergymen who appear to practice medicine by advising certain courses of action, they have little hesitation in teaching their patients and families of patients theology by virtue of their often naïve and ill-formed philosophical remarks in regard to the meaning of life and death. At this point, two courses appear to be open. Either the physician should train himself to be a counselor in the area of morality and philosophical inquiry or he should be sufficiently professional to practice referral to those who do have the requisite training for such guidance.

Any counselor well knows that words of "advice" given to a person in a crisis situation are most apt to be the words of advice taken seriously and since doctors, by the nature of their practice, are constantly thrust into crisis confrontations with persons, they should be well aware that even random remarks at such times carry great weight. One only wishes that most physicians would learn to simply say, "I am not competent to deal with questions of theology or morality. I suggest that we ask for a theological consultation with the chaplain of this hospital or with, if you choose, your own priest, rabbi, or clergyman."

TREATMENT OF CHRONIC ILLNESS—
HOME OR NURSING HOME?

A member of my family has Parkinson's disease and has been in a nursing home for the past few years. Even though I am a physician, I did not fully realize the difficulties inherent in the management of the chronically ill patient until this personal experience occurred. I note with chagrin that clergymen consider visits to a nursing home to be a rather onerous task, and therefore these patients receive less emotional support than I had imagined. It is apparent to me, also, that physicians share this attitude.

The care of the chronically ill patient in all age groups is certainly a major concern in this country, and consideration of the emotional needs of patients in nursing homes will become even more important in the next few years. How does care of these patients, physical and emotional, differ from care of the patient who is acutely ill? What problems are introduced when the patient is cared for in a nursing home rather than in his own home?

RESPONDENT: *F. P. McKegney, M.D.*

Since one in every eleven persons in the United States is sixty-five years old or older, and because great advances have been made in treating acute and life-threatening illnesses, chronic illness is indeed a major problem in this country. In addition, physicians receive little or no formal training in the special problems of patients with chronic or terminal illnesses. Finally, present-day physicians have limited personal acquaintance with death, in contrast to physicians of two generations ago who had, as children or adolescents, usually experienced the death or serious illness of an immediate family member. There is, therefore, an urgent need for medicine to study scientifically the special problems associated with chronic illness, which are quite different from those of acute illnesses, and to develop rational and effective means of treating such problems.

The care of patients with chronic illness challenges the physician's ability to observe, to intervene, and to endure. He must discover the meaning of the illness to the patient and his family. The physician must determine the coping mechanisms and the psychosocial problems of the patient and family which will influence the course of the chronic illness much more than in the case of an acute and curable disease. The chronically ill patient requires more frequent and extensive physical evaluations, because his multiple somatic complaints, though "trivial," may become a major source of anxiety to the patient and of aggravation to those caring for him. The medical care of the chronically ill should be extended to involve resources outside of the traditional doctor-patient relationship. In addition to nurses and social workers, it may be necessary for the physician to involve the patient's family and friends, community agencies, lawyers, and clergymen in the comprehensive care of his patient. Unfortunately, most physicians are neither experienced in sharing medical responsibility nor trained to act as coordinator of a multidisciplinary treatment program.

Early in the chronic illness, there may be great uncertainty, causing the patient and family to ask, "When will it end?" After a variable period of time, uncertainty gives way to hopelessness and the question becomes, "Will it ever end?" To prevent these maladaptive attitudes, the physician must maintain an optimistic relationship with the patient in order to encourage him to trust and to strive for health and usefulness.

Several problems are introduced when a patient is cared for in a nursing home rather than his own home. The strange environment may impair the patient's sense of personal identity and his reality testing ability, causing at least temporary increase in agitation and confusion. The nursing home may engender feelings of helplessness and inappropriate dependency, if more is done for the patient than is actually necessary. The lack of opportunity to carry out familiar activities and usual sources of satisfaction may add to the patient's reaction to his progressive incapacitation.

All of these factors suggest obvious preventative measures. A more complex problem associated with nursing home care is that of the family's guilt over "putting away" the patient. Such feelings have some basis in fact but are frequently compounded by the patient's confused inability to understand and to plan meaningfully and by the emotional tensions between family members which may have little to do with the patient per se. Family guilt should be anticipated and can be modulated or prevented by the physician. He should suggest and arrange discussions between the patient and responsible family members as far in advance as possible of the actual time when transfer will be necessary. A more rational acceptance of this eventuality by all concerned can be accomplished at a time when judgments are influenced less by the severity of the chronic illness or by the urgency of deciding about immediate nursing home placement. Family guilt and the patient's sense of abandonment can be offset by the physician's suggesting a regular arrangement of visits by family, friends, clergymen, and, of course, himself.

Nursing homes obviously vary in their quality, and patient neglect certainly may occur in the poorer-caliber homes. However, there are certain advantages of nursing home care to the patient and the relatives. In the better nursing home, there is probably closer supervision than is possible in the patient's own home. In addition, medical attention is usually more available in nursing homes, especially in those which have physicians who make regular rounds. Most important, in nursing homes the responsibility for care is shared by several people who are less personally involved with the patient. Thus, they are not so drained emotionally and physically as are family members who care for a patient in their own home. The arrangement of private-duty nurses caring for the chronically ill patient in his own home may appear ideal, but it may present certain drawbacks. The expense is considerably greater than for even very fine nursing homes, and the attendance of a physician may be less frequent. Those living in the home of the chronically ill patient are certainly affected by the presence of the patient. Children and adolescents in the home may be particularly affected, especially if the routine of the home centers on the chronically ill person rather than around the lives of the healthy adults and children.

It seems clear that institutional care of patients with chronic illness is becoming a more necessary part of life in our present society. The task before us is to develop means of providing such care which take into account the emotional well-being of the patient and the family as well as the basic physical necessities.

THE MENTALLY RETARDED CHILD

I am a pediatrician who is often faced with the handling of the mentally retarded child. As a physician, I can handle the care and the treatment of the child. The larger problem is that of the parents. What guidance do I give the parents regarding this emotion-packed problem?

RESPONDENT: *Julian P. Price, M.D.*

Dealing with the parents of a retarded child is no easy task. There are no standard rules of procedure. To handle the problem effectively the physician will need, in addition to medical knowledge and skill, an understanding of parent psychology, a desire to be of service, profound patience, and a love for children.

The first essential is the establishment of a diagnosis. This the physician may be able to do from his own examination and experience, or it may be necessary to consult others or even to refer the child to a medical center for detailed study.

After the child's condition has been evaluated, the next step is to inform the parents. This can be an emotion-packed and traumatic experience for the physician and for the parents. To be objective and not appear callous, to be truthful and still offer hope, to express sympathy and not murmur platitudes—of such is the art of medicine. In simple language, the physician should tell what he has found and the conclusions which have been reached. He must be patient and take the time to talk, to answer questions, and to listen.

It is at this time that religious counseling can be of great value. If the physician is a man of religious conviction and knows something of the religious background and beliefs of the parents, he can do much to help these distraught individuals. In addition, a member of the clergy should be called upon—minister, priest, or rabbi—and be urged to work in close cooperation with the parents and the physician.

Finally comes the period of continuing care. The physician should search out the individuals, the agencies, and the organizations in his community which have services to offer the child. Then, with the family, he should help to work out plans for the immediate and distant future. Ever ready to advise and to lead, the physician must be careful not to dictate or to direct. The final decisions regarding the child must be those of the parents.

It is a difficult task, but a most rewarding one for the physician to work with the parents of a retarded child. In what finer way can he carry on the mission of the Great Physician?

RESPONDENT: *Mrs. Malcolm Todd, M.A.*

The physician who is called upon to care for a mentally retarded child must give care in many ways. Physically, of course; but the emotional help given to the parents is certainly of tremendous importance. In order to give guidance to the parents of such a child, it is first necessary to be aware of the dynamics of the situation. How does any parent feel about his child? First, in his child he sees the extension of himself. He is proud; he has certain dreams and aspirations for him. He wants him to be healthy, to excel, to be successful, and to find his place in life. It isn't easy for a normal child born into this world of hope and aspirations to live up to these expectations. It is catastrophic to the parent to have a child born with disabilities that will necessitate a tempering of his fondest dreams, a lowering of his sights, and an adjustment to a new way of life. It is most difficult for the child with disabilities to live in, and adjust to a world that lacks understanding, that is not geared to his disability. Our highly competitive, industrialized, materialistic society tends to disapprove of individuals who will not be able to meet certain standards.

The birth of a child with a handicap places the family in a spiritual crisis and cultural dilemma. How the situation is met

determines whether the family and the child will live together—
in peace, happiness, and security; or in frustration, anger, and
guilt. A birth defect is a family tragedy and in most cases, depending on the severity of involvement—whatever one may do or
say—the tragedy remains. The many emotional feelings—dis-
appointment, anger, guilt, and others—combine to form what
some have called a chronic sorrow. This is an understandable,
nonneurotic response to a tragic fact. The sorrow is chronic and
lasts as long as the child lives. The physician and clergyman concerned with counseling the family must be aware of the emotional involvement. Recognition of the worth of the child, an
attitude of acceptance by society, and patience and understanding
on the part of those who counsel will be of immeasurable help to
a distraught family. Parents often have great reserves of strength.
Acceptance will come in time if parents are helped to deal with
their feelings and if concrete service is available to help them.

The role of the pediatrician is that of a family counselor,
understanding the underlying dynamics of the family constellation with its feelings and emotions. It becomes his obligation to
lead them step by step, toward the goal of increased comfort in
living with and managing a child with a disability.

The physician should acquaint himself with the various facilities in his vicinity for this special child. Public school counselors would be helpful; hospital officials may have suggestions;
public health people could give advice. The National Association
for Retarded Children in New York could be contacted for information. The parent should be made aware of the fact that
thousands of people have faced the same problem and that many
people are eager and anxious to be of help to them in finding
answers to their problems.

ASSISTING THE FAMILY
IN TIME OF GRIEF

I consider one of the physician's major problems to be the compassionate approach to a family when an unexpected death occurs to a loved one. However, I am not certain how this news can best be communicated. What role should the clergyman play and when should he be called in? What guidelines would you recommend in this instance?

RESPONDENT: *William N. Beachy, M.D.*

The principles and guidelines for providing optimum help extend to previous times and circumstances. It is largely a matter of preparation. Most bereaved families will respond adequately to such an agonizing situation if they are given ample opportunity. Those who minister to them must be prepared to bring patience, understanding, skill, and planning to bear upon the situation.

First of all, any who attend the family, and particularly those who deal intimately with them, such as the physician, the nurse, and the chaplain, must understand the reactions of the bereaved. Support through the initial stages of shock, disbelief, emotional outbursts, and clutching at reasons or answers is vital.

Normally it is best to give advance indication that something has gone wrong. This can be done by the nurse, who may ask the family to come to a private place to wait for the doctor who has something to tell them. Although nothing has been said about difficulties, the family will understand that they are to prepare for bad news. When the doctor appears, his demeanor will indicate the gravity of the situation, and using his judgment of the family's reaction, he will first notify them of the patient's death, then answer their questions of how it happened, gradually unfolding the entire nature of the situation as they ask for it.

At about this point it would be natural for the chaplain to appear, unobtrusively making himself a part of the situation in a role which is supportive to the family and to the physician. Together with the doctor, he will, with understanding, absorb the emotional reaction of the family. The attitude of these two persons is the key to the family's ability to understand that they may "go to pieces," and still "get hold of themselves," that they may become angry and unreasonable and still regain their balance.

Proper communication during this period is not so much a matter of what is said, as how this news is communicated. The grief-striken person is largely isolated by shock from his rational faculties. He responds to the emotional tone of the people around him. For this reason those who are to be in attendance must be able to control their own emotional reactions. Suffering, death, human failings, and misunderstandings are all matters to which people can make a constructive adjustment if they recognize them as challenges to be met by faith, hope, and love.

Obviously this degree of maturity and personal capability on the part of the hospital staff presupposes a well-planned, trained, and cohesive community. The hospital administrator bears a large share of responsibility for this. Through his cooperation with the medical staff there can be developed a program of constructive self-criticism which will produce a sense of security in knowing that everything possible is being done to provide the best medical care and to prevent failures and mistakes. Development of mutual respect and support throughout the institution produces a further sense of personal security which in turn provides what can only be described as a healing atmosphere. When this atmosphere exists in a hospital, the entire hospital experience of a bereaved family will support them in their grief. They will not have to battle the feeling that they have been neglected, that there has been no personal interest in them, or that the patient has been just a guinea pig. The nature of the situation is enough to heighten these normal feelings during grief without having them increased by other unpleasant experiences in the hospital. Rather, their almost unconscious observation of the cooperative relationship of all personnel, their warmth, pleasantness, and attentiveness, as well as their skill, will give family members a basic confidence which they will need to draw upon heavily, just as they will receive a major portion of their help from a relationship of friendship and trust with their doctor.

The preparation needed to help relatives during such a crisis results, then, from due appreciation of the principles behind all nonmaterial help given to human sufferers. The general judgment of human nature upon painful or harmful events is that they should not happen. But they do, and if these events are not incorporated into the lives of those who experience them in a positively meaningful way, they cause disruption of personal unity with consequent weakening of the personality structure. This happens when such events are regarded as something to be avoided at all costs and not acceptable in any way. However, they can be incorporated when they are allowed to become the material by which the strength of human nature is perfected. This in turn is possible only when the high value placed upon the individual life resides chiefly in its character. When patience, perseverance, mercy, selflessness, and service are prized, nobility of action under duress ensues. The entire rationale and motivation of service to the sick is founded on this principle. Those who tend the sick do their greatest service in encouraging the sufferer to work nobly with his affliction. Relief of pain and medical or surgical remedies are helps to this end and signs that life and health are worth struggling for. When sickness comes, it is folly to bog down in bitterness at its presence. The attention is turned toward attainment of health. Likewise when death comes, it is folly to bog down in weeping. The character is mobilized to effect a resolution of the grief. When a mistake is made, it is folly to bog down in recriminations and revenge. The attention should be turned to a correction of the cause.

A summary of do's and don't's may serve to illustrate these principles in a practical manner.

Do not try to whitewash the difficulty of pain, suffering, death, human failure, and misunderstanding.

Do not be cold to human grief or unaccepting of the emotional reactions of those who are hurt.

Do not become defensive when at fault, by either denying or downgrading the responsibility, or by seeking too eagerly for expressions of understanding and acceptance.

Do not give the impression of withholding information or hiding facts.

Do not become impatient with the time required to obtain an adequate response or otherwise lose control of your own emotions.

Do not wait for the occurrence of such an event to prepare to meet it, or neglect anything which may be done to assure maximum preparation.

Do not mistakenly conceive that communication is all verbal or that only what is communicated at the time is applicable.

Do not be oversolicitous.

Do face fully the facts of pain, suffering, death, human failure, and misunderstanding, by doing all that is possible to overcome them.

Do rise to the challenge of surmounting your own faults and have faith in all persons to do the same.

Do have more concern for the welfare of the bereaved than for the protection of the institution.

Do depend upon the strength of good relationships with the doctor, the nurse, the chaplain, and others to be a healing influence.

Do make it possible at the right time for the family to become aware of the precautions taken to avoid such accidents and the vigilance exercised to reduce them.

Do remember that the process of adjustment lasts longer than the brief period after death when hospital personnel are with the family. Continue communication through openness to further questions, availability of later reports, and personal attention of high-echelon personnel to final practical details.

Do expand the area of help by fostering the continued care and attention of a clergyman or other supportive person.

CLERGYMEN'S ROLE IN
COMMUNITY HEALTH CLINICS

It is contemplated that a community mental health center will be established in our city in the near future. It is my understanding that experience in other established community health centers indicates that clergy do not refer many individuals who approach them with emotional problems to these centers, or indeed to psychiatric personnel in any facility. What is the explanation for this lack of rapport between clergy and mental health personnel? Specifically, what role do you visualize that the clergy can play in the community health centers? What training is necessary for a clergyman to assume the responsibilities of a chaplain? How can we utilize patient contact with clergy to assist in most efficacious case referral?

RESPONDENT: *E. Mansell Pattison, M.D.*

In the recent national Joint Commission on Mental Health survey, 42 percent of persons with emotional problems reported that they first sought help from a clergyman. They consulted a clergyman usually for a problem of a personal nature in their marriage, with their children, or with their relations. The clergy were preferred to mental health professionals because they demanded less introspection, because interpersonal difficulties were seen more in terms of reality conflicts than psychological conflicts, and because there was less explicit demand for changes in the self. Satisfied with the help they received, people appreciated the clergy for their ability to afford comfort, advice, and reassurance. Most people were not seeking changes for themselves, but were looking for emotional support.

In contrast, only 3 percent of persons with severe emotional breakdowns consulted a clergyman. Because of the severity of their symptoms and the accompanying physical signs, they defined their problem as medical instead of personal and sought medical treatment. Here, treatment for these people was delayed until it was severe enough to draw public attention; or else a long route through various medical and social agencies took them, already severely ill, to mental health facilities.

Although the clergy often see people in early stages of distress, we have not capitalized on their contacts to implement effective early treatment. The clergy make very few referrals (1 percent to 8 percent) to mental health centers. This paradox highlights a problem for preventive intervention where we seek to encourage early identification and referral of the mentally ill to treatment centers.

The problem is twofold. The clergy see many people who do not want to define themselves as ill. People come to the clergyman in distress and will not be content to sit on a waiting list for a clinic or private therapist; many cannot afford even modest fees. Many clergymen complain that realistically they cannot obtain local professional help for their parishioners and so try to "make do." And finally there is still significant suspicion and wariness of an antireligious bias among mental health professionals.

Mental health professionals have been reluctant to accept direct referrals from clergymen. Some mental health centers even have a policy of accepting only medical referrals. Mental health professionals sometimes do not perceive the clergy as professional resource persons, and they transmit a feeling of condescension to the referring clergyman. The clergyman may wish to maintain contact with his mentally ill parishioner during treatment, and this may be viewed as competitive interference by mental health professionals.

Thus, despite the aura of mutual goodwill, I have found little understanding at the grass-roots level. The clergy and the mental health professionals stand wary one of the other, and only in isolated areas have effective means of collaboration, referral, and treatment programs been established throughout the country.

The clergyman with special clinical training may fill four main roles in the program of a community mental health center. These roles range from the traditional pastoral role to that of "religious expert" consultant to the total program of a center.

1. *As a director of pastoral care.* This function involves all those usual religious activities which clergy provide: religious services, administering the sacraments, making individual pastoral calls, etc. These may have generic and specific values. The chaplain has a responsibility to the entire patient population and to the therapeutic program as a whole. As such, he can implement religious programs which may not necessarily have specific theological aims but are primarily therapeutic in intent. We might call this "generic religious activity." In addition, the chaplain may provide specific spiritual services or arrange for visiting clergy to provide specific sectarian rites.

2. *As a consultant in psychotherapy.* Here the chaplain functions in his pastoral role, but with a primary concern to assist in the treatment process. He may (a) counsel on theological and religious questions, (b) offer appropriate support during periods of anxiety, (c) help the patient fit his religious background into his therapeutic experience, and (d) engage in religious rituals appropriate for problems of sin and guilt.

3. *As a diagnostic consultant.* Here the chaplain functions not as a clergyman but as an expert on religious matters. He may explore the patient's religious life with the expert knowledge of various religious cultures and the role of religion in the personality. The consultant then develops relevant additions to the psychodynamic formulations of the patient's problems and recommendations for the appropriate use of religious resources in the community for rehabilitation of the patient.

4. *As a liaison to the religious community.* Here the chaplain moves into a role which capitalizes upon his clerical identity, religious knowledge, and contact and identification with the religious community. He can provide education and consultation to the community mental health team and the clergy of the community, interpreting each to the other. The need here is for a chaplain who is thoroughly familiar with the treatment of the mentally ill and with the resources of the community. He must

be able to communicate easily and meaningfully with psychiatrists, psychologists, social workers, and others on the mental health team as well as with his fellow pastors.

A chaplain in a community mental health center must have specialized thorough training in the mental health field. Such training should enhance his professional skills as a pastor, but it should not be focused on psychotherapy. He should be an expert on mental health, but not someone interested primarily in doing some kind of individual therapy himself. He is, in fact, a fellow member of an interdisciplinary team. Such training is now available in accredited training programs of one- to two-year duration in many hospital and mental health facilities. These include didactic courses and supervised clinical experience.

The key to utilization of the clergy as community resource persons lies with the mutual education of the clergy and mental health professionals in their respective collaborative roles. Many mental health centers now offer ongoing consultation to the clergy of their community and employ trained chaplains on the professional staff to assist in the type of liaison described.

RELIGION AND PSYCHIATRY:
A POLYGON OF RELATIONSHIPS

Paul W. Pruyser, Ph.D.

In a vague way, relations between religion and psychiatry are
as old as civilization, but that observation is as troublesome as
it is edifying. For instance, the fact that ancient temple healings
of the mentally deranged in Egypt, Greece, and Rome are on
record says little more, after some reflection, than that ritual
played an important role in ancient medicine, as it did indeed
in all walks of life. The twelfth-century report of a Jewish
traveler who visited Dar-el-Maristan, an asylum for the insane in
Bagdad kept up by the caliphate, is intriguing as an instance of
religion's concern for the mentally ill, but loses some of its charm
when one hears that the patients were chained to the walls in
manacles. Upon hearing that in the fourteenth century some
European monastaries opened their doors to the care of lunatics,
one will rejoice, until one discovers that the regimen for the
patients differed little from the daily routine of the monks, in
which the whip was a prominent instrument.

There may be more comfort in knowing that in 1408 the
first European asylum for the mentally ill was established in
Valencia, by the church. Healing of mental illness was also
sought at shrines of special patron saints, out of which grew
eventually the still famous therapeutic community of Gheel in
Belgium. But Luther advocated the drowning of mentally retarded children and much of the splendid sixteenth and seventeenth centuries linked mental illness with demoniac posses-

sion, with treatment appropriate to that diagnosis. Should we consider the *Malleus Maleficarum* of 1480, that manual for exorcists and religious torturers, a landmark in the relations between religion and psychiatry? Or should we choose the year 1564, when Johannes Weyer published his *De Praestigiis Demonum*? He fulminated against misplaced culpability in cases of demon possession, pleading for a humanitarian understanding of the poor women who were thought to be devil's helpers or who themselves claimed to have sold their souls to that influential gentleman. The answer will depend on how one sees the relations between those two human enterprises and what aspects of these one will admit or omit. Certainly, the long historical look shows that healing and worship can tumble into superstition, stupidity, and cruelty; that both can make the same error; that one can criticize or improve upon the other; and that either or both can be helpful in promoting human welfare. Both enterprises have sometimes shown very similar manners and sometimes strikingly different ways.

But should not one first define religion and psychiatry? By all means, if the days of one's life are plentiful enough to try it. For our purposes it is more important to know that the words "religion" and "psychiatry" are both quite complex designations, pointing to forms of knowledge, types of practices and skills, social institutions, value orientations, professional roles, academic disciplines, and whatnot. They are not spatial realities like areas or fields or realms, of which one could discuss boundaries or regulate the traffic patterns. They are, rather, specialized perspectives in which to apprehend and influence all the very complex realities of human life. Each of these perspectives has its own history, its own fundamental assumptions, its own methodology, its own cognitive and operational goals, its own failures and successes.

A second point of some importance is that each of these perspectives has a theoretical and a practical aspect. Each also contains basic science of a sort and has an applied practice or skill aspect. Moreover, there is much contending in the relevant professional circles about the relations between the basic-science and the applied-science aspects of each; indeed, some outsiders have even raised a question whether the term "science" is appropriate at all to the two groups of disciplines. At any rate, one should from the outset acknowledge tensions within each perspective: psychiatry is not the same as psychology, sociology, medicine, anthropology, or popular ideas about mental hygiene —although it has much to do with all of these; systematic theology is not the same as pastoral theology, pastoral care, Hebrew, excavations, or popular statements of belief—yet it has much to do with all of these in ways which are harmonious and embarrassing. My use of the words "religion" and "psychiatry" will always imply recognition of these inner tensions within the two perspectives.

Recent History and Beginnings of Structure

As to the history of relations between religion and psychiatry, I will start at a point where these become articulate, interesting, and productive. Nearly all of this history is recent, beginning around the turn of this century. As long as psychiatry was really neurology or merely an esoteric pastime of classifying, it had little relevance to religion. And as long as the faithful defined religion exclusively in terms of the supernatural or lustily thought of detachable souls floating through a never-never land, with God having spoken once and for all in the King's English of the seventeenth century, there was no need for any conversation with psychiatry. I think it is defensible to say that the history of relations between religion and psychiatry begins with two epoch-making changes: (1) the stirrings of the psychodynamic point of view in psychiatry, launched and epitomized by Freud, and (2) the upswing in various schools of biblical text criticism, led by Wellhausen and widely known through Schweitzer's *Quest of the Historical Jesus*. Added to these was the profound concern with religious *experience,* opened up for scientific inquiry by psychologists of religion and students of phenomenology and comparative religion, so popular in the first few decades of our century and led by such men as William James, Rudolf Otto, Frazer, and Jordan. I also wish to note the contextual influence of the social gospel movement, Bushnell's renewal of religious education, and the ecumenical movement.

In dynamic psychiatry there is a long line of development, from Freud's early studies, through his friendship with Oscar Pfister, a Swiss clergyman and psychoanalyst with whom he corresponded for three decades, to *The Future of an Illusion,* published in 1927, which gives a thoughtful functional analysis of the uses of religion in life. Of many other important studies there is only space to mention the work of Theodor Reik on ritual. In religion there was an equally vigorous concern with sociological analyses of church life, with reflections about interim ethics and the Kingdom of God on earth deduced from new understandings of eschatology. To all of these trends on both sides the notion of development became ever more crucial, whether it meant the long-range developments of historicism and phylogeny or the short-term developments of ontogeny and social engineering. Both parties had a new respect for natural law and empiricism.

In this setting we find one episode that was to have *organized operational implications* for both disciplines: the mental illness, in the early 1920's, of a Protestant clergyman who asserted that some severe mental disorders may entail a profundity and lucidity of experience closely akin to, if not the same as, the states of religious insight reported by men of acknowledged religious genius. I am, of course, speaking of Anton Boisen who eventually published in 1936 his *Exploration of the Inner World,* after having laid the groundwork for what is now called clinical-pastoral training through experiments in Worcester State Hospital. He was greatly aided in this endeavor by Richard Cabot of Boston and drew near to such leaders as Healy and Bronner, Helen Dunbar, and others at Harvard, Union Theological Seminary, and Chicago Theological Seminary. The new hospital chaplaincy, thus inaugurated, was no longer a pious window dressing for poorly run state hospitals, but a new and disciplined form of ministry which had healing as a coordinate goal and required the idea of a diagnostic and therapeutic collaboration between psychiatrist, social worker, chaplain, and nurse (the psychologists came on the scene somewhat later). It helped in bringing about the beginnings of psychiatric team practice.

Meanwhile, the psychiatric professions continued their clinical interest in the study of mental processes, such as motivation, the function of conscience and values, the role of ideals, the aberrations of wishful thinking, and the important question of developmental stages and crisis. As psychotherapy and milieu treatment came in greater use, many old academic questions received new clinical answers. Distinctions were introduced between healthy and unhealthy religion, between regressive and progressive religious themes, between defensive use of religion and conflict-free religious ideation or practices. From the other side, the new clinically trained chaplains were able to make fresh observations about religious psychopathology and maturation, which greatly enriched the traditional, normative psychology of religion. Indeed, they tended to relocate the laboratory of that discipline from the university campus, with students as the typical guinea pigs, to the mental hospital, with patients as the typical sources of data. They also added a social dimension missing in most psychiatric thought of the time, namely, that illness and the hospitalization process are a crisis situation for patients and families, needing a sacramental approach celebrating the idea of community, much as religion had traditionally done with birth, death, confirmation, bereavement, and marriage. The expanded view of the ministry now included, with new technical competence, the ill, the bereft, the deranged, and the criminal.

These intertwining strands had theoretical and practical implications. Psychiatry and psychology became more and more a basic science to theology and pastoral care. A new interest was awakened in "images of man" more empirical than the old doctrines of man, enriched by clinical observations, personalistic and process philosophies, and new pastoral practices. A new perspectival view was in ascendance, particularly in theology itself, which renounced the false comforts of splitting reality neatly into natural and supernatural realms, separating the disciplines into sacred and secular concerns, and wrapping knowledge into revealed and profane packages.

There was also an increasingly sophisticated mutual assessment between the two perspectives. I will mention only Roberts, Hiltner, and Outler as leading minds among many who, while deeply grateful to psychiatry, also threw a theological searchlight on its theories and practices, at times exposing the cryptotheologies of psychiatric thought. Similarly, there were psychiatrists who were concerned over the cryptopsychiatries of pastoral work and the psychological naïveté of some theologies. Again, I have space to mention, among many leading men, only Menninger, Zilboorg, and Bartemeier, who also felt that psychiatric training should include instruction about many religious phenomena and practices.

All of this had the effect that pastoral theology, which had sat for some time rather meekly at the feet of a psychiatric Gamaliel, rapidly turned the relation between religion and psychiatry into a two-way pattern. This reciprocity resulted also from newer developments in systematic theology which took the psychiatric disciplines seriously, lending them respectability by transposing psychiatric theses into philosophical categories and vice versa. The work of Tillich has been very important in this regard, and I am tempted to include also the influence of Bultmann, whose demythologizing has at times a psychological ring.

In the 1940's and 1950's, much work went into the development and acquisition of psychological skills among practicing pastors. Under the influence of Rogers, Curran, and Wise, the pastoral counseling movement began to blossom; the hospital chaplaincy developed increasingly sophisticated supervision techniques and case methods for teaching, while the practice of group dynamics and group work began to be applied in large segments of church life. Basic psychodynamics, clinical psychology, and psychopathology slowly began to replace the importance of educational psychology in the seminary curriculum. A generation of pastors and theologians had emerged with sufficient psychological knowledge and clinical experience to enter peer-level dialogue with the professionals in mental health. Interdisciplinary conferences were held, such as the Gallahue Conferences at the Menninger Foundation and the Arden House Conferences of the

Academy of Religion and Mental Health, which demonstrated responsible conceptual inquiry, a willingness on both sides to pool knowledge and resources, and an eagerness to engage in respectable exchange of ideas and experience.

A final word needs to be said about the role of existentialism in articulating some relations between religion and psychiatry. An existential concern has marked most Protestant theology of this century, has influenced pastoral activities to a large extent, and has been inherent in the development of dynamic psychiatry. As a matter of fact, phenomenological methods are important in religion and in psychiatry, and have at times provided a common basis of approach to the data of experience. The various existentialisms, however, are something else. In psychiatry, many of them skirt clinical issues in favor of some sort of metapsychology or even philosophy; in theology, some promising, open-ended existential leads have turned into prematurely closed systems. Nevertheless, it seems to me that the language and topical interests of some existential writers have functioned as a bridge between theology and psychiatry and have enhanced the possibility of dialogue, even when they have had little effect on psychiatric and pastoral techniques.

The Role of Communication

In the polygon of relations between religion and psychiatry, adequate communication is, of course, of vital importance. The two different perspectives involve two different language games, imply different meanings in common words, and value the various aspects of communication differently. Risking overstatement, I am tempted to say that, in psychiatry, expertise in listening is more highly prized than skill in speaking; in theological circles the opposite values prevail. If one takes a long look at the many articles, books, and speeches which have been published on issues between religion and psychiatry, one cannot help feeling that much writing has remained uncommunicative, while some of it has been outright solipsistic, clannish, or parochial. It is indeed not easy to strike the proper tone that is heard unambiguously by friend and foe alike or to find the proper level

of conceptualization accessible to professionals from both perspectives. I am sure that this had to be learned, for the published
literature does show a marked progress in this respect. Special
journals such as the *Journal of Pastoral Care, Pastoral Psychology,* and the *Journal of Religion and Mental Health* have
brought about increased sophistication and more efficacy in communicating across the different disciplines.

Two dangers lurk here. The first danger is to find easy comfort in similarities between the two disciplines pitched at too
high abstraction levels. As a rule, the higher one moves up the
abstraction ladder, the more one finds a forced likeness between
things after having stripped away their individuating features,
so that one ends up in the syncretistic position that everything
is basically like everything else. This process not only falsifies
reality but puts an end to the fascination of inquiry and dialogue. The other danger is to stay so close to raw observations
and simple activities that theoretical formulations are held to
be of no account. My own preference is to proceed, with some
humor, with comparisons at a relatively low level of theoretical
formulation, acknowledging the ad hoc or fragmentary nature
of most theories in all disciplines and shying away from over-
indulgence in metapsychology. I find some of these desiderata
satisfied in Hiltner's *Preface to Pastoral Theology* and Erikson's
Young Man Luther, strikingly flouted in most Jungian studies
and nearly impossible to get across to strict Barthians.

Professional people have their own specialized vocabularies
which can be misused as a status symbol, a weapon, or a secret
language. These can also give a false security to their users,
feigning knowledge where there is only speculation or opinion.
For these reasons, mere versatility in the use of the other man's
technical terms cannot be taken as a reliable sign of adequate
communication between the two disciplines. Instead, it may be
a sign of arrogance, intrusion, or defensiveness.

Goals and Means of Religion and Psychiatry Relations

Relations between religion and psychiatry can be grouped
into theoretical and practical ones, in terms of goals, methods,
or operations. Many of the early contacts were initiated by re-

ligionists, interested in acquiring psychiatric knowledge in order to achieve the end of more purposeful pastoral work through more efficient skills. Similarly, many of the current relations between the two disciplines are initiated by psychiatrists, also for very practical ends. When the report of the Joint Commission on Mental Health and Illness stated that 42 percent of all people aware of having a personal problem first contact their minister, rabbi, or priest for help, it behooves psychiatrists to recognize that pastors serve in our society as frontline mental-health workers, playing a vital role in secondary prevention, and perhaps in primary prevention as well. The training of ministers in psychological knowledge and skills, commensurate with their pastoral role, thus became a vital concern for the mental-health professions, and accorded with already existing desires in many clergymen.

Other relations stem from concerns with theoretical formulations and conceptual inquiry between the two disciplines. Psychiatrists and psychologists may have an interest in psychology of religion, in group life in churches, in religious education, and in administrative structures of churches. Even if they had no such interests spontaneously, they may be asked to give advice or consult with ministers or church organizations regarding such matters. Similarly, ministers and hospital chaplains and theologians may take an interest in the interactions between social ethics and psychiatry, the vocational and career stresses of workers in the mental-health professions, the overt or covert religious assumptions made by some psychiatrists, or the philosophical tenability of certain theories.

In the practical collaboration between religionists and psychiatrists one should distinguish between working for psychological goals and working toward pastoral goals. Sometimes these goals may be coordinate or parallel; sometimes they merely require similar or parallel activities; but whatever is done or striven for, in however different or similar fashions, the professional roles in which the activities are carried out will always be different, with different language games, with different symbols, and under different ultimate auspices.

Since both groups of disciplines are immensely complex,

meeting grounds between them can sometimes be better provided by a third discipline than by a direct confrontation of the
two. I think that sociology, cultural anthropology, ethics, lin-
guistics, and philosophy have often mediated between the two
parties. In addition to academic interactions, however, there are
the practical social problems such as marriage and family life,
sexual ethics, delinquency and crime, civil disobedience, and
many urban problems linked with rapid social change which
often bring about practical cooperation between religion and
psychiatry even when the theoretical frameworks taken abstractly
would seem to preclude any fruitful sharing.

Roles of Models and Constructs

Organized thinking tends to take a selective focus on a limited situation, a delineated problem, or a special metaphor.
Thought in religion thus tends to be organized around liturgy,
proclamation, various doctrines, care, and the congregation.
Thought in psychiatry may be organized around hospitalization,
diagnosis, psychotherapy, special forms of psychopathology,
methods of treatment, etc.

It seems to me that in the recent history of relations between
religion and psychiatry there has been a selective use of some
models, with the neglect of others. Much has been made of various models of illness and health, often under such topical head-
ings as "sickness or sin," "anxiety and the fear of God," "pain
and suffering." These involve exceedingly difficult questions not
only between the two disciplines but within each of the two. A
purely organically oriented psychiatric nosology will give one
answer, a descriptive psychopathology another, a psychodynamic
point of view a third, and so forth. Various theologies will define sin, the fear of God, or suffering in strikingly different ways.
Small wonder, then, that explorations of these broad topics are
rather unrewarding as long as they are allowed to remain global.
Useful discussion of models must be more precise and limited.
Discussions of "sin and sickness" will not get anywhere until
they have become articulated into something like "the concept
of sickness in Freud's later period compared with the concept of

sin in Calvin's *Institutes*." While this sounds like the title of a doctoral dissertation and may have little appeal to the general reader, it is nevertheless the stuff that respectable studies are made of.

One prevailing model for explorations between the two disciplines has been psychotherapy and counseling. An enormous number of books and papers has been written about these, and while many of these have been rewarding, some have perpetuated a lopsided view of what most psychiatrists do most of the time. Psychotherapy is only one among many treatment methods, and large amounts of psychiatric work are more comparable to first aid, management, advice-giving, and teaching than to the "thorough overhaul" of personality which is the popular view of psychotherapy. Perhaps the greatest single psychiatric function is diagnosing. Certainly a large part of psychiatry is hospital management, and it seems to me that this model of the theory and practice of managing a hospital or a ward could be a very fruitful model for ministers who are in the business of "managing a church."

The consideration leads to the next model: the question of solo practice vs. group practice or teamwork, in psychiatry and in the church. I believe that one of the most outstanding features of psychiatry is the organized teamwork between members of several disciplines in the service of healing the sick. The team is not an organization chart or merely a set of coordinate roles—it is far more unique and subtle than either of these. It is a delicate process of maintaining and suspending certain professional prerogatives, keeping alive creative tensions about one's identity and roles, and using one's specialized talents for thinking in interdisciplinary terms. An exploration of the team model may be of great benefit in considering the ever growing trend toward multiple-staff ministries (with and without specialization) in the churches and the recognized difficulties in relating the various levels of church organization to each other.

Another promising model, on which some work has already been done, is the nature of the community in hospital and church. What are the actual operations of such communities?

What is their ethos? What are their goals? How do they come about? How can they be balanced between organized structure and spontaneity of formation and functioning? How does one move into and out of such communities? What does it mean to minister within the hospital community and what does it mean to practice so-called community psychiatry in the open situation of town and city? Obviously, the idea of a community is complex; it requires multidisciplinary study and will undoubtedly be a useful model for continued explorations in religion and psychiatry.

Parenthetically, it is interesting to note that ministers and psychiatrists, roughly at the same time in history, have begun to display some impatience with confinement to the pulpit, the hospital, and the office, and are seeking ways into the open community for new professional challenges. While both groups have always been deeply involved in helping to bring about meliorative changes in individuals under their care, they are fast becoming also agents of change in the social and cultural currents of our time. I think this being an agent of change is another fascinating model with vast implications for theory and practice.

Some New Frontiers

The forward thrust of history always leads one to consider the future in the light of what was and is. Can something be said about possible new frontiers in religion and psychiatry? I think there are some hints about the shape of things to come and I will simply enumerate them, without quite knowing how and when they will be realized.

In the first place, I see a good deal of movement taking place in theological education, in the general direction of bringing into the seminary curriculum some of the historical assets of training in medicine, law, and the social sciences. I think there will be more emphasis on fieldwork for pastors; more utilization of theories and techniques of close supervision during the practicum years; more use of the case method; more demand for firsthand experience with the whole network of caring and helping agencies of the modern community; more deliberate exposure to members of other healing, helping, and caring professions. While some of these features are already present in quite a few seminaries, they are too often seen as an alien oddity rather than as an integral aspect of the education of ministers.

A second frontier seems to shape up in regard to the study of religious experience and conversions. This is really an old interest, shared by such men as James, Boisen, and Jung, but the possibilities for a truly experimental approach to it have only been opened recently by the advent of such pharmacological agents as lysergic acid diethylamide (LSD), psilocybine, mescaline, and similar compounds. While the work being done in this field is still controversial, it is likely that an increasingly better control of all the variables in such drug-induced states may be reached which will undoubtedly advance the scientific status of the findings.

I believe that a third frontier needs to be developed, even though there are as yet few signs of lively interest. It will consist in the application of psychiatric and social theories and techniques to the religious mission field. Most mission boards still favor surgeons and internists and specialists in tropical medicine in the medical missions, overseas and in national mission areas. This preference has been and still is defensible, but it is becoming ever less cogent in view of the tremendous social changes occurring in the so-called less-developed countries, in which mental-health problems, identity crises, shifts of habits and loyalties, rapid cultural change, social-mobility problems, and explosive aggressive reactions and depressions are the order of the day. Since church missions are part of these social changes and like to think of themselves as having been a contributory cause as well, it would behoove church boards to give fearless thought to the relevance of psychiatry to mission work and apply for help, at theoretical and practical levels.

At this day and age I should end on an ecumenical note. It has been astounding and rewarding, in my own experience, to see how constructively clergymen of different denominations and faith groups can work together when they focus on common problems. Some of the newer thoughts on the pastoral ministry, the nature of the church, the meaning of symbols, and the hazards of communication have been fertilized by psychiatric ideas. I am sure, although it is rarely admitted, that some of the new thoughts about community psychiatry have been fertilized by ideas derived from the pastoral ministry. One of these is the exploration of techniques of helping persons or groups who have not asked for help. The mutual influences of these models and the interpenetration of great ideas have not only fostered goodwill and understanding between religion and psychiatry, but have also, in the hospitals, clinics, and helping agencies, enhanced cooperation and unity among responsible leaders in the denominations. In this sense, the work of Pope John XXIII not only announced a new prospect but summarized what had already taken place. For this reason his name belongs in this sketch of a polygon of relationships between religion and psychiatry.

SEX AND
THE PRACTICING PHYSICIAN

William F. Sheeley, M.D.

Since ancient times and before, people have turned to the
family physician for help with problems affecting their sex lives.
Although they may not say so unless he encourages them, they
expect his help to understand the perplexing and often terrifying
emotions which they feel in themselves and observe in others.
Parents ask him to explain to an adolescent son "the facts of
life" of which they themselves are not too sure even after years
of marriage. Or the son himself haltingly asks the doctor to explain the alarming things going on in his body and in his
thoughts. Couples bring to him problems blighting their marriage bed. Other people question him about fears that they are
perverted, weak, or diseased.

These sexual problems are often not as simple as they seem.
They may be but the overt show of many hidden conflicts. The
complexity of these problems is not surprising, for they stem
from forces which pervade most of the physiological, psychological, and social aspects of the person. Sexual feelings and activities,
whether normal or disordered, are the final common pathway
of a complex constellation of numerous and various influences
and conditions. Sexual feelings and activities certainly have roots
in physiological function. But they also have roots deep within
the psychological being of the individual and within his interpersonal adjustments with other people. They are affected by
strivings for power, by longings for dependency, by fears of

abandonment, by threats to life itself, and by feelings of pride and self-esteem. People use the promise, the giving, and the withholding of sex to bribe, dominate, cajole, disarm, mollify, ward off, frustrate, reward, mislead, reassure, exploit, and comfort others.

Little wonder, then, that one who closely examines a given sexual problem may discover behind that problem somatic or psychic disorders. Behind the impotence of a man or the frigidity of a woman, one may find depression or alcoholism or an anxiety state. But one may also find diabetes, carcinoma, or adrenal tumor. Behind a man's flagrant sexual behavior—such as exhibitionism, child-molesting, or homosexuality—one may find schizophrenia, severe personality disorder, or brain tumor. Behind a young couple's loss of their erstwhile delight in sexual intercourse, one may find a family breakdown—a breakdown in urgent need of attention. Behind a man's inability to assert his masculinity in bed may lie an even greater inability to assert himself in the competitive world which surrounds him and his family.

Although sexual problems may arise from somatic disease, then, they much more often arise from psychosocial disorders, for sex is an individual and a social affair. Sexual activities concern people singly and in pairs, true, but they also concern society at large. Laws and social customs governing marriage and divorce reflect this concern. That basic unit without which few societies can survive—the family—depends upon discipline and control of sexual behavior. Without such control, the family soon breaks down, and soon thereafter the whole society comes crashing down—like the mighty Roman Empire, which is no more.

No society has solved the problem of providing, on the one hand, great sexual freedom for its members and, on the other, adequate safeguards to protect and care for the children which issue from sexual activity and upon which the society's continued existence depends. The individual who follows society's official dictates and the one who defies them fail to adjust, each in his own way. The prim old maid is an object of general scorn; the philanderer, one of contempt. True, most societies provide subtle devices for the individual to violate surreptitiously the overt social code without attracting public wrath. But these devices are, at best, unsatisfactory. In the end, each person must solve for himself the problem of meeting the demands of society and of his own nature. The solution is not easy. Attempts to find a satisfactory compromise create conflict, emotional upheaval, and suffering. Little wonder that so many people flounder into complicated messes, and then turn to the family physician to extricate them.

For example, sexual drives and angry feelings often blend, or one takes on the qualities of the other, so that one activity is used to express a feeling to which it is not logically related. The man who rapes to vent his anger at women or at the world, the woman who strips off her clothing before a hundred men and then goes home to sleep with her girl friend, the man who writes a dirty book which makes sex organs and sexual intercourse repulsive, the wife who chastises her husband by denying herself to him, the husband who responds to his wife's sexual invitations with impotence, the teen-age girl who eats her budding young figure into a revolting blob—all of these can have, and usually do have, the common denominator of hostility, which has somehow gotten mixed up with sex.

The family physician is potentially a most valuable case finder of sexual problems among his patients. As we have already noted, part of his value as a case finder stems from the fact that people tend to look to him for help with those sexual problems of which they are very much aware. A woman who has not yet read her Kinsey, for instance, believes that her husband's "depraved" sexual foreplay is a sickness and therefore sees her doctor about it. A man comes to him for a fancied magical pill for his impotence or for his wife's frigidity, which he ascribes to a somatic cause. Still another patient brings symptoms, such as headache, backache, fatigue, or general weakness, which he ascribes to anemia or another purely somatic cause; he has no inkling of the pathogenic sexual disorder.

But if the family physician is to realize this great potential as case finder and as healer of sexual disorders, he must have more knowledge about normal and abnormal sexual practices than he likely has today. He must have sufficient knowledge to determine whether a given set of sexual disorders arises from predominantly somatic causes, from psychic causes, or from a combination of the two. He must know how to help his patients and their spouses achieve adequate sexual adjustments. To do so, he must know how to guide and counsel them when the solution of their problems lies primarily within themselves, and he must know how to treat effectively those sexually related psychiatric disorders which are within his therapeutic competence. In this connection, he must know how to judge which of these he can correctly treat himself and which he must refer to a psychiatrist. He must know how to anticipate and how to prevent the emotional trauma of sexual maladjustment between the bride and her groom.

By and large, neither medical schools nor other sources of sexual knowledge available to the physician have prepared him adequately to assume these responsibilities. The physician's own sexual experience, however amusing and remarkable when recounted in cocktail lounges, may hardly equip him for his counseling tasks. When he tries to discuss sex with his patients, therefore, his offerings are likely to emphasize the anatomy and physiology of the sexual organs. These are important, of course, but they have little to do with the really troublesome aspects of the whole matter. They leave quite unanswered difficult but pertinent questions: Why? When? How? The physician may adopt a posture which is either too strict or too lax morally—or too different in quality from the patient's own moral code—for the patient to accept it. His own problems in this sphere may intrude into the therapeutic process. He may become so uncomfortable and embarrassed that he makes the patient equally uncomfortable, so that they both then seek the cool relief of changing the subject. Or he may permit himself vicarious pleasure which the patient soon detects, and the patient flees from this "too nosey" doctor. In any case, the patient's problem remains unsolved.

Many physicians, then, need broader and deeper education about sex with particular regard to its importance in medical practice. To meet this need, medical schools and training hospitals, in their undergraduate and graduate curricula, should devote sufficient attention to the subject to give the physician entering medical practice the confidence of sound knowledge and the poise of professional objectivity. Since sexual problems permeate all of medicine and are not the exclusive concern of psychiatry, instruction should relate them to all the fields of medicine. Certainly the obstetrician and gynecologist, as teachers, should include the effects of sexual problems in their discussions of such conditions as dysmenorrhea and infertility. Proctologists should underscore the importance of reassuring the patient facing prostatectomy as to the expected sexual sequelae of the operation. Cardiologists should instruct the student as to what limitations, if any, a cardiac patient should place on his sexual activities and encourage the student to provide answers spontaneously to questions which the worried patient will not bring up for fear of embarrassing himself or his physician.

In the meantime—until medical schools have filled this gap, and for the sake of those physicians who have left medical school —there must be offered programs of continuing education which broaden the practicing physician's knowledge and skills dealing with sexual problems among his patients. Until teachers in other medical fields have themselves developed greater interest and knowledge in this aspect of their fields than they presently have, it may be wise for practicing physicians to look to the psychiatrist for such continuing education.

Psychiatrists, it is often true, have themselves neglected the relationship between sexual difficulties and specific somatic illnesses and situations. But they have had some explicit instruction in the field, and in their daily practices they grapple constantly with the sexual concomitants of psychiatric disturbance. It is therefore reasonable for the practicing physician to turn to them for educational programs, and it is fair for him to expect them to heed his request.

Sexual problems cause great misery to individual men and women, to husbands and their wives, and indirectly to their children and to others with whom they work and otherwise associate. The family physician has many unique opportunities to help relieve that misery. Properly equipped, he can take advantage of those opportunities and he and his patients will profit.

SEXUAL EDUCATION FOR ADOLESCENTS

An earnest young Protestant seminary graduate has come to be an assistant minister in our suburban community. He wishes to undertake some sort of sexual education of the adolescent young people in the church, before they encounter the sexual temptations which are bound to arise in high school and college. If he undertakes this task in cooperation with one of the physicians in the congregation, what should be the role of each? Is it necessary to obtain the consent of the parents of the young people before such counseling is undertaken?

RESPONDENT: *Truman G. Esau, M.D.*

Clergymen and physicians frequently collaborate in programs of sexual education for adolescents in the church. This has become a common pattern and is a commendable one. It is doubtful however that the participants always realize the depth of the issues they are touching. First, one must differentiate between the importing of sexual information which can be done in an academic manner and sexual education which aims at altering emotional attitudes. Such a goal cannot be accomplished in one evening's session nor is it realized simply by using "the right techniques." The clergyman and physician must have a grasp of the dynamics and the interpersonal relationships with which they are dealing when they open up this important and sensitive subject. It can be emphatically stated that no such program can alter the emotional attitudes of adolescents with regard to sexual material unless the family is touched as well. This stems from the fact that the psychosexual growth and development of moral and ethical structure in a child is not a matter of having correct information, sufficient warnings, or vivid illustrations. Sexual attitudes are not simply an expression of what one knows, but are formed within the matrix of the child's exposure to his parents' marriage. So such a presentation is not dealing with the isolated need of an adolescent but with a family process. As a consequence, it would be wise for the parents to be involved from the start in such a task. It would be good to enlist key parents in the early preparations for development of such a sexual education program. Their leadership can do much toward gaining acceptance and support within the congregation. Consent need not be obtained from each parent for the young people to be involved in such a program if the leadership adequately prepares and informs the parent group prior to such meetings.

Above all else the important mood to be achieved in such programs is one of honest confrontation. First this necessitates openness of the clergyman and physician to each other. If they do not understand their goals, their prejudices, and commitments, anxiety will interfere with their cooperative venture, resulting in subtle clashing or avoidance of conflictual areas. Consequently it is best that the clergyman and physician be well known to each other and share a high degree of mutual respect of each other. This honest encounter first between the clergyman and the physician must then be carried forth with the adolescent himself. The purpose of the meeting is not simply to provide sexual information, although such information is necessary and may serve as a vehicle of open discussion. The purpose of the meeting is to give the young person permission to listen, to participate with his peers and with the leaders, and to share his ideas as he desires.

Traditionally there has been a division between what is presented by a clergyman and what by a physician. It has been common for the physician to start such a meeting with a presentation of basic physiological and anatomical material. It would be well for the physician to remember that most adolescents have long since gained this sexual information and are frequently well aware of sexual anatomy and physiology. This is gained early in life because of an exposure to peers and the increasing openness in our society about sexual matters. What must be remembered even more is that adolescents have not necessarily gained proper emotional values with respect to this information that they have learned. So the tone of respect, value, and purpose that the physician places upon sex will say as much as the content that he is presenting.

It has been common for the clergyman to present next the moral and ethical issues. One serious deficit that has characterized many such collaborative ventures has been the ignoring of the interpersonal family relationships which are so critical in the development of sexual attitudes. The proper preparation, and especially the use of a series of meetings rather than a "one-night stand," may well be able to capture the trust and stimulate the group to discussion of the personal and family dimensions. Neither the physiology nor the morality of the sexual material presented need be the primary message. Of greater importance will be the interpersonal focus upon the subtleties of affection, the sharing of emotions, and marriage as represented in each family. It is not uncommon, when adolescents are exposed to such a situation, to talk freely about the problems in their parents' marriage, masturbatory conflicts, questions of sexual expression among themselves, etc. It is best that such panels and group discussions of sexual material focus upon the rich meaning of sex in human life. The primary purpose of these meetings is not to attempt to constrain the young person, although certainly moral and ethical issues are properly raised. It is rather to give the young person a setting in which he can understand and approve of his own feelings and also gain encouragement to develop the controls that are necessary for the development of honest, secure, and stable personal relationships for the present and in the future.

The leaders should feel the freedom of organizing the group as they wish, by dividing the sexes or combining them. It would certainly be beneficial, if tolerable for the group, to invite the parents to participate in some phase of the discussions. This would likely be a much more stressful type of meeting, one aiming at the creating of some bridges where there has been distance and suspicion between the adolescent and his parents. The clergyman and the physician may need to structure this meeting more definitely because of the high level of anxiety in the adolescent and the parental group. However, honest expression of feelings is essential here also.

Subsequent to such seminars, the clergyman and the physician should be aware that they are now in a special position in the eyes and feelings of the participating adolescents. They should remain available for appropriate counseling as requested by adolescents from the group. They may also need to refer some to more specialized persons in the community. Exposure of severe family problems, serious sexual preoccupations, or persistent sexual deviancy are indications for professional psychiatric help.

THE ROLE OF THE SCHOOL AND THE COMMUNITY IN SEX EDUCATION AND RELATED PROBLEMS

Thomas E. Shaffer, M.D.

There is a universal feeling that not enough nor the right kind of sex education is being done at home, in the school, or elsewhere. Most parents, teachers, physicians, ministers, nurses, youth leaders, and school and college youth would agree that there could be improvements.

Sex education is a complex topic. There is, however, as we all know, more to it than classroom instruction, because under this "umbrella" are a number of related but individual goals. Among these are answering simple questions of children; supplying facts about the anatomy and physiology of the organs of reproduction; providing help and direction to boys and girls in establishing appropriate masculine and feminine roles; developing acceptable sexual behavior; preparation for marriage; a foundation for responsible parenthood and achievement of a happy, stable family life; comprehending the issues in population controls; teaching the importance of preventing certain infectious diseases; and reducing the problems of premarital pregnancies, abortions, and illegitimacy.

I do not attempt to solve all of these problems in the general subject of sex education during this discussion. According to Sidney P. Marland, Jr., Superintendent of Schools in Pittsburgh, one "powerful force now emerging in the 1960's is a spirit of inquiry, change, experimentation, and critical thinking." [1] It is in this current of thought that I, a physician, discuss a matter of concern to all of us.

Inadequate teaching. Signs of inadequate teaching about sexuality and family living are numerous: unhappy people, disorganized homes, divorces, irresponsible behavior, and inability to discuss the subjects of sex and reproduction plainly and without embarrassment. The reason for this appears to be that teaching reproduction and sexuality is a cooperative endeavor involving, at various times in a child's life, the home, the school, and other resources in the community. Truly, all of us are dealing with some aspect of the problem in our own ways every day. No matter how sincere the people who deal with children at specific ages or times may be, there is bound to be some impairment of the end results of disorganized, unrelated efforts.

Today's infants are the adolescents of tomorrow and the parents of the near future. What we do for the benefit of school children is not, therefore, solely for their immediate needs. We have an opportunity to prepare them for their future roles as adults and parents. Thus, I see sex education as applying to an endless series of stages in life, a continuum from birth through childhood, adolescence, young adulthood, to parenthood, and as the circle closes, to the birth of a child in the next generation. Parents, educators, and physicians may stand in relation to this situation like the blind men, each of whom described an elephant from the particular part he could feel, failing to appreciate the qualities of the whole beast.

Instruction for adult responsibility. The logical place to start in this discussion would be with the needs of an infant. This would indeed comfort this pediatrician who is, in fact, none too confident at this point. But infants have parents who play an essential role in the early life of their children. Most parents cannot perform this part well by ear, so let us first start by considering opportunities for preparing people and especially adolescents for the eventual responsibilities of parenthood. This would indeed complement adolescents' drives for independence and for acceptance as adults. Instruction for an adult responsibility might be more palatable than "sex education." Some background of factual information about reproduction acquired by them earlier in life must be assumed. This is reasonable, for reproduction education is the basic component of sex instruction in most schools. There are many other grounds for sex education which too are a function of schools, but we will come back to them when the hypothetical infant grows older and enters school.

Optimal development of the personality, attitudes, and feelings of children and youth depends on achievement of the developmental tasks of infancy and the preschool period. This stage of life necessarily takes place in the home under the good or bad guidance of parents. The best-intentioned parents usually lack information, vocabulary, and naturalness to carry out the all important early sex instruction of their children. Some feel inadequately prepared. Some feel modest or embarrassed. It is not really difficult theoretically to answer the simple questions of a three-, four-, or five-year-old about his body, reproduction, and sex differences. But, because this phase of our education was usually not handled adequately a generation or so ago, we, the parents of today, have carried over the attitudes of our own parents.

The learning of facts about reproduction and sexuality and the capability to tell others about it must come from opportunities in the high schools and programs for parent education in the community or in the schools. No matter how novel, organized, and different, future approaches to sex education in the schools may be, they will be less than ideal if children enter school with no information about sexuality or with the wrong kind, and with well-established, but unfortunate, attitudes and feelings that reproduction and sexuality are naughty, vulgar, and not to be mentioned in public. Early experiences, especially those in the home in the formative years, leave lasting effects on personality. According to Eisenberg who was discussing the permanence of early impressions and experiences, "Whether or not appropriate 'experiential supplements' during adolescence can lead to successful negotiation of this period despite pathology in earlier life is not known." [2]

Obviously, some of the most significant information and attitudes are gained years before teachers and others serving young people have a chance to influence them. We do not have a favorable opportunity later on to affect social behavior, promiscuity, venereal disease, illegitimacy, and the other problems we talk about in connection with sex education unless a child has a fairly good start in a stable, affectionate home environment where, among the favorable things, sexuality is treated in a frank and intelligent way. Such a start will not be easy to bring about, nor will it be as successful as we would wish it to be because education for parenthood is not easily accomplished. According to Brim the eight important groups engaged in parent education in this country—family life educators, medical personnel, nurses, clinical personnel, home economists, clergymen and religious educators, teachers, and parents who have received special training—have not conclusively shown, in evaluation studies, that they change parents or children by any of the usual methods of mass media, individual counseling, or group discussion.[3] We who work with children at a later age must accept this challenge to get at the very roots of emotional and social ill health. One of the ways to do this is to give older adolescents and young adults a suitable vocabulary for teaching their own children in a comfortable, frank fashion. The second phase, learning the essentials of child development, will enable them to assume the first stages of sex education during the preschool years.

Approaches to sex education. Some of us learned a few years ago at the University High School in Columbus, Ohio, that teaching of this kind could be done when it was planned to be objective and impersonal.[4] A child health conference was conducted in the school during the regular school day, so that high school pupils, in a coeducational situation, could observe the conference and discuss subjects which are normally embarrassing. Reproduction, pregnancy, the process of birth, the care of the infant, and growth and development were discussed in as much detail as the pupils wished, using appropriate vocabulary. There was absolutely no tension or embarrassment. Countless frank and unexpected questions were asked of the mothers or the nurse and pediatrician by the students without hesitation. Of course, one reason may have been that the physician, nurse, and teachers were more comfortable and confident in this situation, rather than the probability that the student lost his discomfiture in his interest in what was taking place. It will be necessary in the spirit of inquiry, change, experimentation, and critical thinking to search for more of these situations and to develop them for practical, meaningful teaching.

Remember that Thomas Parran, M.D., in 1936 when he was surgeon general, started a successful campaign to remove secrecy from venereal disease and bring it into the open for discussion and understanding. We are faced with a somewhat similar situation with respect to education about sexuality. Our goals are education about reproduction and sexual behavior and in addition, vocabulary, self-confidence, and ease in dealing with these subjects.

Not all children, by any means, will receive desirable or even acceptable care, affection, and education in the home from their parents. Many of them will have a deprived infancy and childhood, often with one, sometimes with both parents out of the picture. Often such children come under the influence of some agency in the community, perhaps a day nursery, a public health well-child conference, a church school or some other child care unit in which concern for the development of sound ideas about their sexuality could be developed. If these opportunities are not seized upon, the result will inevitably be that children will search on their own for information later on and they will not find informed persons for this. Sometimes they never cease searching or as we call it later on, experimenting. Seldom will they develop wholesome attitudes this way.

A child's quest for information. There is good evidence that uninformed children and adolescents most often obtain their sex information from the peer group rather than from parents or counselors. In a school health education study it was ascertained that among ninth-grade students, "when bothered with a sex question three-fourths of the boys and one-half of the girls indicated that they would never, or only sometimes, turn to either parent or school counselor for information." [5] There are reasons to believe that the ones who do turn to reliable sources are the ones who received frank, simple, straightforward answers to their questions early in their lives.

Children reach the kindergarten and first grade in a stage of latency as far as psychosexual development is concerned. During the period between five or six years and nine or ten, there are occasional requests for factual information about reproduction and anatomical differences. The children who missed out on early, wholesome learning experiences at home are the ones who are the problems, as they come with unsatisfied curiosity and false information. They can be identified and deserve special attention from teachers. Breckenridge and Vincent give some help in this regard in stating ". . . by the time children enter school they should have adequate words for the eliminative processes, should know the true origin of babies, and should be familiar with the differences between boys and girls." [6] This is a guide for parent goals and for teachers. Newly developing programs like "Operation Head Start" provide a special opportunity for getting closer to mothers and young children. Parent education for these disadvantaged families is one of the requirements. What a novel chance this is for schools and other institutions and agencies to get in "early licks" never before so attainable! These are the people most in need of motivation and professional help.

One of the developmental tasks of childhood which must be accomplished is the creation of one's sexual identity and appreciation of the social role of one's sex. Normally this comes about within the family through children seeing the culturally recognized role functions of each sex and by emulation of the parent of the same sex. Outside the family this sex-role identification occurs in association with one's peers. Through observing and reacting, the child becomes aware of what sex he is and what is appropriate behavior. This is not an automatic outcome, because in some homes there is only one parent, perhaps of the opposite sex. Other environmental conditions interfere. It has been said that appreciation of sexual identity threatens to become a cultural problem in the United States where father may be in the kitchen wearing an apron and doing the dishes while mother is mowing the lawn, garbed in pants.

Is there not an opportunity for others who come in contact with children outside the home to play a part in establishing appropriate sex roles through activities, assigned duties, teaching and example, and requirements for dress? An example of an adverse trend is a query received recently by a medical group from some educators for advice about the safety and the appropriateness of touch football as a sport for girls in schools and colleges. Acceptance of one's own sexual role and one's sexual behavior is probably more dependent on learning than on hormones, assuming of course that adequate physiological maturation has taken place. There was a rousing ballad in the musical *Flower Drum Song,* entitled "I Enjoy Being a Girl." The stanzas of that ballad go further than I have in explaining the sum and substance of these remarks.

The latent period of development comes to an end with the first signs of pubertal growth and development. Questions about one's body again become of top level priority and this time with a difference: the questions now have a direct significance for "ME." It is essential to anticipate this need of ten to twelve-year-olds by being ready with an educational program whether in a course or discussion groups. The need and the opportunities are found in the early, not the later, period of adolescence.

Werkman lists the following as adolescent crises: body changes, dating, identity challenges, and maturity.[7] Parents contribute to these emotional upsets of adolescence by "increasing the sexual concerns of adolescence." Their own views and example are paramount. Of course, the example and stimulation of press, radio, and films are a large factor in creating turmoil. In these early adolescent years, when sexuality is first appreciated, help from outside the home is needed. It is easier to direct and nurture attitudes at this time than to try to change the mores later on. We are now at a time of considerable change in sexual codes among young people which will not be discussed here. In the early adolescent years children want some direction and preferably from sources outside the home.

The number of normal adolescent children who become concerned about whether they are normal is greater than those who really have something to worry about. The facts and mechanisms of adolescent growth and maturation must be explained before anxieties develop. This entails teaching about the variations in time, amount, and pattern of pubertal development. All children will not be satisfied or reassured easily. There will always be those who fear they will not grow or that they will not stop growing in height, breadth, and among the girls, in those important three measurements recorded for Miss America contestants.

Our experience in a medical clinic for adolescents has consistently shown that worries about variations in growth or maturation are a major cause for seeking medical advice. Most of the problems are not organic abnormalities, for they fall within the range of normal variation. However, they are important to the adolescent at the time. Preparing children in advance for such variations is preventive medicine in practice.

Children in the preadolescent years have no great concern for themselves—what they are, what they look like, and what they will become. The adolescent years are different, with strong drives for independence from parents, status with peers, and socialization with the other sex. The net result is an increasing concern for one's ability to succeed in these areas and to be successful eventually as an adult. Without opportunities to talk about his concerns, an adolescent may develop an image of himself as inadequate and become socially isolated from his peers.

"High-risk" children. In obstetrics and pediatrics there is an effort to identify those women who, for various reasons, are most likely to deliver infants who do not live or are below par if they survive. Research and specialized medical care are being concentrated in this "high-risk" group of women for the purpose of using medical resources to the best advantage and being ready for problems when they occur. There are, among children, those who might be classified as high-risk in respect to the needs of their emotional and social development.

These high-risk children with respect to needs, attitudes, and behavior are first of all the ones who enter school with inadequate knowledge and warped views about sex. A simple, obvious example is an "only child" or even one with no sibling of the opposite sex. Others in this category are ones who for some reason are not accepted by peers or at least feel that they are not. These children, sometimes transplanted from rural area to city or from one part of the country to another, perhaps outsiders because of socioeconomic differences, or ones with physical handicaps, are likely to be the ones who isolate themselves. Later they may join a "crowd" or form a too-strong heterosexual attachment (going steady) which could lead to a pregnancy, an illegitimate birth, or a too early marriage, and usually the end of their academic education.

We are concerned today about the rising incidence of venereal diseases, the out-of-wedlock pregnancies, illegitimate births, and teen-age marriages and divorces. There is no need to enumerate statistics or to point out the unwelcome results of these events. There are definite opportunities to influence these trends by facts and by nurturing rational attitudes and acceptable behavior. It will not be simple, because there are cultural, social, and educational forces which interfere. I am not certain whether the basic philosophy should be to consider these situations as representing irresponsible sexual behavior or as being the result of lack of knowledge or indifference. I could not agree with a public health "adviser" who is quoted as having said with reference to a television V.D. education project he described as a "scare method." "We want to be falling just a little short of panic in the streets. . . . If the nation has got to have a phobia, it might as well be a syphilis phobia." [8] On the other hand, it is impossible to accept a view that "Our young people are drifting into and establishing a new permissive code of sexual behavior— one in which they will eventually find happiness and adjustment with behavior patterns that ridicule premarital chastity and the sanctity of the marital relationship." [9]

Conclusion. We are at a crossroads. We can go on much as we have for the past several decades, teaching about reproduction and sex, attempting to instill good values in children who come to schools with those values, good or bad, already quite firmly established, and hoping to control irresponsible behavior by facts and by fears of V.D. and pregnancy. But if we really want to accomplish the goals, we must have foresight, more wisdom and imagination, and more results. One of the signs of change in this direction is the formation of SIECUS (Sex Information and Education Council of the United States), a new organization, which "expects to work closely with established, family-centered, interdisciplinary organizations to help bring about, within the framework of family life education, constructive dialogue between youths and adults on the pros and cons of the various sex patterns that can be identified in American life." [10] I recommend this council for information in the coming years.

It may well be that sufficient respectful attention has not been given to thoughtful views of adolescents themselves on the subject of sex education. Calderwood has written a stimulating and fascinating account of his work with a group of high school youths in Oregon along these lines. The goals these young people listed, after many individual and group sessions with their skilled, understanding leader, provide a challenge to any group or individual affecting sexual education:

1. To provide whatever factual information the individual desires on all aspects of sex.
2. To increase self-understanding so that individuals may become self-confident members of their own sex.
3. To increase understanding of the opposite sex in order to promote positive relationships between the sexes.
4. To understand better other patterns of sex behavior among peers, among the adult generation, and in other cultures, so as to prepare individuals to live with others who believe differently.
5. To open up communication and promote understanding between adults and youth.
6. To develop an appreciation of sex as an integral part of life and see it in the perspective of one's whole life.
7. To allow and enable each individual to develop a personal standard based on understanding of and concern for others.
8. As a continuous process to prepare individuals mentally and emotionally for their biological development through maturity.[11]

SEX AND MENTAL HEALTH ON THE CAMPUS

Seymour L. Halleck, M.D.

There is general agreement that sexual attitudes and sexual practices in American society are undergoing radical changes. I propose to examine the extent of these changes and to describe their impact upon the mental health of university students. My approach while hopefully not moralistic will not be free of value judgments. Like most psychiatrists I consider mental health to be something more than mere adjustment to the needs of the community. Mental health is defined according to certain values, values such as psychological comfort, intimacy, compassion, social responsibility, and self-knowledge. Once the psychiatrist begins to ask if a given sexual behavior is good or bad for a person's mental health he is no longer in a position to avoid making ethical judgments.

How much change has there been in sexual attitudes and behavior among university students? Recent surveys suggest that there have been important changes in students' attitudes toward premarital sexual intercourse. These changes are most apparent when student attitudes are compared with those of their parents' generation. In one study when adults were asked if they believed sexual intercourse would be acceptable if a couple were engaged, only 20 percent of adult males and 17 percent of adult females said yes. In a student group, 52 percent of the males and 66 percent of the females answered the same question affirmatively. In another study, mothers and their co-ed daughters were asked to respond to the question "How important do you think it is that a girl be a virgin when she marries?" Of the mothers, 88 percent answered very important, 12 percent generally important, and 0 percent not important.[1] In a preliminary study of sexual attitudes of freshman and sophomore girls at the University of Wisconsin, Dr. Richard Sternbach and I found that only 30 percent felt that premarital intercourse was definitely wrong.

In judging the rightness or wrongness of premarital intercourse, today's student is confronted with alternative value systems which he can either accept or reject. Most students feel free to search for a morality which suits their own needs. They are not necessarily contemptuous nor rebellious toward older generations. Rather, they have a live and let live attitude. Students often say, "I wouldn't feel bad if I participated in premarital intercourse, but I wouldn't want my parents to know about it because they would feel my behavior was wrong. What they don't know won't hurt them."

Attitudes toward discussing sex have also changed. In the past two years, members of the University of Wisconsin Department of Psychiatry have had many requests to speak to student groups about sex. We have all noted an amazing openness and frankness on the part of male and female groups. Seventeen- and eighteen-year-old girls for example have little shyness in a group setting in asking speakers about such previously taboo subjects as masturbation, orgasm, techniques of intercourse, oral-genital relations, and homosexuality. All students seem to be eager to create a dialogue with older generations as to the pros and cons of premarital intercourse.

Although there is undoubtedly a revolution in attitudes toward sex, accompanied by a refreshing frankness, there is nevertheless little evidence that the actual rate of premarital intercourse has radically changed. It may be true that more and more young people are engaging in heavy petting before marriage. But the physical state of virginity still seems to be the norm. Kinsey, studying volunteers, found that from 1910 to the 1950's there was no appreciable increase in the proportion of girls having intercourse before marriage.[2] More recent depth interview and questionnaire studies of randomly selected populations at major universities suggest that approximately four-fifths of undergraduate girls have *not* had coital experience.[3] At the University of Wisconsin, for example, a 1966 survey of three hundred freshman through senior girls indicated that only 22 percent had experienced sexual intercourse.[4]

We might assume that some day the actual behavior of students will more closely approximate their expressed attitudes. Nevertheless, as of this date there is no evidence of a radical increase in premarital intercourse among university students. It may be reassuring in this regard to note that the great majority of students do not condone promiscuity. When they insist that premarital relations are morally justified, they are most frequently referring to intercourse between those who are engaged or deeply in love. Very few girls can envision themselves having relations with more than one partner. Of the ninety girls Dr. Sternbach and I surveyed, only four defended sex as something to be casually enjoyed with several partners. Some behavioral scientists believe that our culture is moving toward the Scandinavian model of sexual behavior which condones premarital sexual relations between people in love.[5] The expressed attitudes and actual behavior of our students reinforce this notion. In other words, it is unlikely that we will become a promiscuous society, but it is quite likely that we are on the way to becoming a nation in which couples who intend to marry begin sexual activity before marriage.

A trend toward sexual permissiveness based on affection and love should not alarm psychiatrists. After all we believe in the values of intimacy and compassion, and the new sexuality seems to be moving in that direction. Unfortunately, the problem is not that simple. If a girl accepts the new attitudes and wishes to have sexual relations with a boy on the basis of mutual affection and love, she must still define the strength of their commitment. Inevitably she must struggle with the question of how close two people can be when not bound to one another by the responsibilities of a marital contract. Any relationship out of wedlock is plagued with certain ambiguities. The girl must struggle with questions such as, "Will the first argument or sign of incompatibility lead to a dissolution of the relationship and a search for a new partner?" If this does happen, will she simply deceive herself into promiscuity under the rationalization that each new relationship is meaningful? Will she "kid herself" into believing that she is in love when in actuality she is only succumbing to social and sexual pressures? It is my belief that these ambiguities have been heightened by changes in attitudes toward sex. The stresses associated with choosing or sustaining sexual relationships before marriage have had an especially intense effect upon female students. For some students such stresses have been critical factors in precipitating severe emotional disorders. In this sense a significant number of students are casualties of the sexual revolution.

Mental Health and Sexual Permissiveness

If it is true that rates of sexual intercourse before marriage have not changed appreciably in the general student population, this trend is not apparent in those students who are psychiatric patients. In a recent survey of twenty-four Madison psychiatrists who were treating University of Wisconsin students, I found that of their one hundred and seven unmarried female patients 86 percent had had sexual relationships with at least one person and 72 percent had had relations with more than one person. Permissive sexual activity seems to be highly correlated with mental illness, or at least with a willingness to accept a mental illness role. This data raises some disturbing thoughts. Psychiatrists and other physicians have been in the vanguard of either praising or deploring new trends toward permissive sexuality. Judging from their publications, it appears that psychiatrists have gained the impression that promiscuity is rampant in our youth. However, if we compare the incidence of virginity among nonpatients with that among patients (remember that only 22 percent of the nonpatient students had had sexual intercourse) it appears that psychiatrists err when they generalize from experiences with a somewhat atypical clientele. Patients may be promiscuous, but most of the population is not.

How can we understand the relationship between mental health and permissive sexual behavior? Is it possible that casual sexual behavior can cause girls to be mentally ill? Or does being mentally ill make one more susceptible to free and easy sex? Or does some third factor have a causative influence upon permissive sexuality and mental illness?

There is certainly a great deal of support for the latter two hypotheses, particularly for the proposition that poor mental health makes one more susceptible to frequent sexual contacts of a promiscuous nature. Martin Loeb has noted that teen-agers who trust themselves, who can contribute to others, and who can rely on others tend to have the least number of sexual relationships before marriage.[6] Maslow has described the sexual behavior of very healthy "self-actualized" people and notes that they have fewer premarital sexual contacts than less successful people. Their attitude seems to be, "We don't need sex but we enjoy it when we have it." Maslow points out that self-actualized people enjoy sex more than others but consider it less essential in their total frame of reference.[7] My own observations of highly disturbed delinquent girls suggests that their promiscuity is determined by primitive neurotic needs and is only one symptom of a pervasive emotional disturbance.[8] These girls seek multiple sexual experiences because they have despaired of finding any other means of obtaining nurturance and affection.

It is also possible that a high concordance of sexual permissiveness and mental illness is related to a third factor such as urban sophistication. Conceivably those who are most willing to accept psychiatric treatment are part of an avant-garde who are also willing to enjoy an unrestrained sexual life. Still another possibility is that a willingness to be a mental patient and a willingness to be a casual sexual partner are related to a general sense of alienation. An increasing number of students have rejected the prevailing norms of their own cultures and have not found substitute moralities with which to identify. Such students may be exceptionally casual about sex, and the painful effects of their identity diffusion may then be likely to bring them to psychiatrists.

Granted that mental illness may lead to promiscuity or that a third factor may be related to both, to what extent is it possible that liberal sexual behavior might be a *cause* of mental illness? Here we must be wary of circular thinking. The lower classes of society are willing to define promiscuity as "badness," but many members of the middle and upper classes automatically define it as "illness." The social conditioning of an upper or middle class girl leads her quickly to accept the patient role once she begins to think of herself as promiscuous. Sociologists and anthropologists might argue that there is no causative relationship between permissive sexual behavior and mental illness but that society simply equates promiscuity with mental illness as a means of enforcing chastity. They would insist that if permissiveness were the norm, promiscuous girls would not be patients.

The sociological argument is partially correct. I believe, however, that promiscuity can still produce emotional problems and that its causative influence is in practical terms relatively independent of current social definitions of normative behavior. The experiences associated with being promiscuous are in themselves stressful and are not conducive to the development of those personality traits generally considered to be characteristic of the "healthy" individual. Furthermore, whether society is right or wrong, it does impose social stresses upon the promiscuous girl which are sufficiently painful to drive her to the mental illness role.

I have noted that those students who are patients have a greater tendency toward promiscuity than the average student. It must be acknowledged of course that not every female patient who has had one or several affairs should be considered promiscuous. However, the kinds of stresses such students experience and the manner in which these stresses drive them toward a patient role will be clarified if we consider the case of one highly promiscuous girl.

Joan, an eighteen-year-old girl, made a psychiatric appointment the morning after she had slept with the tenth different boy in the space of a year. Sensing something self-destructive about her behavior, she made a pledge to seek help after her tenth affair. She had been depressed and unable to study. Her school performance had deteriorated to the point where she was contemplating leaving school. Joan initially had doubts about accepting the role of patient. She defended her sexual behavior, insisting that it was correct and moral. Although she assumed her parents would not approve of her conduct if they knew about it, she derided their values as "phony" and insincere. She maintained that she had experienced orgasm in every sexual encounter and that each new affair was more exciting than the last.

During the first month of treatment, Joan added two more lovers. When the therapist asked what these affairs meant to her, she stated, "It's just fun, like eating a good meal or seeing a good movie. The boys mean nothing to me; they just enjoy me, and I enjoy them." During this time her school performance continued to deteriorate. She smoked marijuana, drank heavily, and increasingly talked about the meaninglessness of life. As she became more depressed, she began to voice thoughts about suicide.

In the twelfth hour of therapy, the patient reported that she had recently slept with a boy whom she actually despised. She was agitated and remorseful. At this point she began seriously to review her sexual history. She had had her initial affair one year earlier with a boy she had thought she loved. When he broke up with her, she had three new experiences in rapid succession. In each case Joan tried to convince herself that she was in love with her boyfriend, and in each case her relationship terminated in less than a month. Joan then decided that she would never sleep with another boy unless their relationship was meaningful. The next three relationships however did not last more than a week. Two of the boys did not even bother to call back after the first date. As Joan related the rest of her history she tearfully stated, "The last few months I've just been kidding myself. I try to convince myself that I really love these boys, but really I'm just scared that if I don't sleep with them no one will even ask me out. I begin to hate myself, but I can't stand the loneliness."

Joan was fortunate in having a successful therapy experience. Eventually she was able to feel better, to improve her school work, and to find a boy whom she married. One interesting aspect of her therapy was that after a year of treatment and after she had found a boy who loved her she admitted that she had previously never experienced orgasm during coitus. At this point she wondered how she could ever enjoy sex with anyone but her fiancé and admitted to considerable remorse over earlier sexual experiences.

While I was convinced that Joan's personality problems had made her susceptible to promiscuity, it also seemed clear that her promiscuity had contributed to a state of chronic despair. As with so many girls, Joan's initial intention to associate sex only with love was subverted after the first few affairs. Eventually, sex became for her a remedy for loneliness. Her belief that she was finding intimacy and meaningfulness through sex was painfully recognized as a self-deception. It is difficult to see how Joan could have found intimacy or love. Her relationships were simply too transitory. There was no opportunity to get acquainted with her lovers. At the first argument, the first feeling of disgust, or the first incompatibility, separation loomed as the most seductive alternative.

Joan's misery was at least in part related to a pervasive sense of guilt about her sexual activities. A sociologist might argue that Joan's guilt was caused by her restrictive upbringing and society's puritanical attitude toward sex. Indeed, Joan accepted this argument and insisted that her guilt was extraneous to her, a foreign body imposed upon her by a malevolent and self-righteous society. As an impersonal act, sex is a vehicle for expressing any type of emotional need humans can experience. In addition to being a source of physical pleasure, the sexual act also fulfills dependent needs, status needs, and aggressive needs. Psychoanalysts (particularly Bergler, Brenman, and Reik) have pointed out the way in which the quest for gratification of such needs comes to be associated with feelings of guilt.[9] The girl who uses sex to combat loneliness, to gain status, or to exploit others cannot avoid a certain amount of guilt. Even if she is able to free herself from religious or moralistic scruples, she must deal with those guilt feelings which are associated with the selfish or aggressive uses of sex.

Furthermore, any dishonesty in the sex act, such as pretending to love while not loving, pretending to be someone else, pretending that her partner is someone else, or even pretending to enjoy the act while not enjoying it, can lead a normal person to feel guilty. The partner who constantly feels that she takes more than she gives will also be uneasy. So will the person who uses a moderately deviant fantasy to stimulate her sexual interest. In this day and age we have even invented new guilts, namely, guilt for being unattractive or guilt for not having orgasm. It is unlikely that even the marriage contract does much more than attenuate these feelings. It would seem that all of the kinds of guilty feelings I have described are more likely to occur in a promiscuous relationship. To the extent that a girl such as Joan accepts the new sexual attitudes and actively seeks sex without guilt, she deceives herself and runs the additional risk of feeling more guilty simply because she knows she *is* guilty.

Another adverse effect of promiscuity which is apparent in Joan's case is that more sexual freedom for women has not been accompanied by an elevation of their status as women. The double standard is still with us. I have never heard a single phrase from any student, male or female, which suggests that girls were more esteemed as important and worthwhile persons because of their enlightened sexual attitudes. At the same time, I have seen many patients who abandoned career aspirations once they began to be involved with multiple partners. Unfortunately the sexually permissive girl comes to see herself as more of an object and less of an equal partner. At the same time, she is given more responsibility than ever before for prevention of pregnancy and is probably less able than girls of previous generations to count on the help of her boyfriend if she is impregnated. In effect, she is valued by men for her sexual capacities and for these alone. Social conditions may of course change, but the present trends toward sexual permissiveness have not liberated women, they have only strengthened the feminine mystique.

We might also note that a repetitive break with the rules of society pushes the promiscuous girl closer and closer to alienation from society. As her self-esteem declines and as she becomes more accustomed to rule-breaking behavior, she desperately seeks rationalization for her conduct. These are most easily found in attacks upon the entire social code. An overdetermined attack on the beliefs of the older generation moves the promiscuous girl further away from her own past. She begins to lose perspective on that part of her own history which identifies her with her society. Such alienation is highly correlated with feelings of powerlessness, with abdication of responsibility and, ultimately, with a willingness to identify oneself as a patient. Some of these problems are closely related to an increasing tendency of our youth to live in the present, to deny fidelity to past values, and to despair of hope in the future. Promiscuous sex contributes to such tendencies by its immediacy. It calls for gratification "now" and denies the possibility of better days ahead. Very few promiscuous girls look forward to a better sexual relationship after marriage. While it is difficult to determine which causes which, promiscuity is usually linked with alienation and seems to encourage withdrawal from social responsibility.

May has defined Puritanism as a separation of passion and sexuality.[10] May believes that the old Puritans were passionate but not sexual and that many of our students are new Puritans in the sense that they are sexual but not passionate. Certainly in the case of Joan and other promiscuous girls, it is difficult to find the kind of passion and commitment that is characteristic of deeply involved people. The new sexuality does seem to be frighteningly sterile. An emphasis on orgasm pervades all age groups in our society. Among university students, the search for the ultimate orgasm has become almost a competitive matter. In Joan's case, it took over a year of therapy before she could admit her relative virginity. In our age, this has become the ultimate confession. I have seen other girls who admitted cheating, stealing, masturbating, and promiscuity with little shame but who wept violently when they confessed that they could not have orgasms.

While promiscuous girls emphasize the importance of orgasm, they are often too immature to actively desire or enjoy sexual intercourse. They are ahead of themselves in the sense that they could enjoy intensive petting, but actual coitus is perceived as alien and frustrating. One of my promiscuous patients stopped taking her birth control pills because of medical problems. Knowing that she could not have intercourse without risking pregnancy she settled for heavy petting on her next date. During an intense petting session she experienced an extremely satisfying orgasm, the first she had ever had outside of masturbation.

The stresses of promiscuity are indeed intense. Not only is the promiscuous girl denied intimacy and plagued with guilt and alienation, but she is often limited in her capacity to feel physical pleasure. Furthermore, she feels obligated to convince herself that she does experience pleasure and is likely to be guilty if she does not. If she feigns orgasm, her guilt is even greater.

The Borderline Girl

Let us now leave the problems of the promiscuous girl and consider the girl who believes that intercourse before marriage is morally justified only if it is always associated with love and commitment. What pressures does such a girl wrestle with, and how are these pressures related to her mental health?

In lengthy question and answer sessions following informal talks to female students, I have become convinced that the new sexual attitudes are having a significant influence upon all female students. More girls may not be indulging in premarital intercourse, but more girls feel pressured to do so.

The mass communication media in our country have a tendency to emphasize the most extreme forms of social behavior and to present them as the norm. Our students receive a heavy bombardment of *Playboy* philosophies which argue for the enjoyment of sex for the sake of physical pleasure alone. There are few social forces counteracting these philosophies. Even our religious leaders are modifying their pleas for rigid adherence to premarital chastity. Our youth seem to have accepted a number of questionable beliefs which serve to perpetuate these pressures. For example, many of the girls I have spoken to believe that physical frustration per se is psychologically unhealthy. They are convinced that petting without orgasm will be unhealthy for them and their partners. They continue to believe that there is an erotic health-producing quality to orgasm during intercourse which is not available through masturbation. While this belief is not supported by any current research, it nevertheless continues to exert a powerful influence.

Many girls also fear that denying their sexual charms to boys is a sign of selfishness. In an age where students are deeply concerned with communicating and cutting through one another's defensiveness, the act of intercourse is valued as an easy means to such goals. Not infrequently, the girl who retains chastity is accused of emotional coldness, of not trying to be an open person. Finally, most girls believe that there is more sexual activity taking place than is actually the case. If they do not participate, they see themselves as atypical and strange.

There are other highly varied pressures which produce conflict in the girl who wishes to make a rational decision as to premarital intercourse. Many girls simply feel that they will lose their boyfriends if they do not sleep with them. Others have convinced themselves that technical "know-how" is important for a successful sex life and that experience before marriage will make them better wives. Finally the Vietnam conflict has had a deep impact upon people of draft age. Some girls out of guilt, compassion, or love feel obligated to give themselves to those who could lose their lives. The phrase "Make love, not war" is a political slogan, but in this day and age, it is also an effective argument for sexual permissiveness. All of these pressures produce conflict in the girl who wavers between chastity or fidelity and greater sexual freedom. Sometimes the conflict is directly related to the development of psychiatric difficulties.

Barbara, an eighteen-year-old freshman student, came to the clinic because of nervousness, depression, and inability to study. She was unable to sleep, had lost weight, and was becoming increasingly preoccupied with the meaninglessness of life. Barbara had received a Fundamentalist Protestant upbringing with strict sanctions against premarital sex. In spite of this, she had engaged in one prolonged and satisfying affair with her high school sweetheart. She had hoped to marry the boy, but he eventually rejected her.

In the course of her first interview, Barbara revealed that she had been assigned to a dormitory with girls who took a decidedly casual attitude toward sex. Her closest friends, including her roommate, were all promiscuous. She suspected that her friends were emotionally disturbed people, but she liked them and she was deeply impressed by them. As the semester progressed and Barbara learned more about her friends' sexual activities, she began to question her own values. She had always had a strong need for group identifications and a wish to be an "in" person. When her friends chided her as prudish, old-fashioned, and selfish she felt despondent. She was tempted to sleep with boys, but her early upbringing made it impossible to adopt a liberal attitude towards sex without experiencing enormous guilt. Faced with such conflicts, she became increasingly anxious and depressed. By the time she came to the psychiatrist, she was beginning to move toward withdrawal and alienation.[11]

It can be argued that Barbara was an immature girl who would have had difficulties irrespective of the social climate or her fortuitous association with promiscuous dormitory mates. I am not convinced. In a different era, or even in a different dormitory, Barbara's conflict would have been less intense. She had been exposed to a social climate in which the pressures for liberal sexuality were as great as or greater than the pressures for chastity. She was not experienced enough nor had she developed a sufficiently stable identity that she could resolve her conflict by selecting a value system which was congruent with her own sense of self.

Not all girls, of course, are as intensively exposed to subcultures of promiscuity as Barbara. Nevertheless, this subculture does exist on our campuses, and its influence is greater than would be anticipated from the size of its membership. Promiscuous girls are often seen as representing the vanguard of a new and better morality. They are not looked down upon by chaste girls (although interestingly enough, they themselves are quite contemptuous of those who are not promiscuous). Newspapers, periodicals, and television describe them as the "new breed," as the "now people," and impressionable youngsters take these images seriously. In such a climate premarital intercourse can be enforced upon a girl in a manner not too dissimilar from that in which chastity was enforced upon girls in an earlier generation. Under such pressures, many girls like Barbara experience intense conflict which cannot be resolved without psychiatric assistance.

The Problems of Virginity

Psychiatric problems associated with efforts to retain virginity are not too different from those seen in the past. Psychiatrists still see patients whose depression and psychosomatic disorders appear to be directly related to repression of sexual drives. Of course the pressures against virginity are greater today, and a girl may have to develop rigid and highly maladaptive defenses if she wishes to remain chaste. Virginal girls are also tempted to exploit men into committing themselves to a more permanent relationship. This is especially true among those girls who espouse an "everything but" philosophy, who engage in heavy petting but stop at the point of intercourse.

Perhaps a new trend is indicated by a few girls who come to psychiatrists and present virginity as a problem. Such girls accept a moral code which condones premarital intercourse but find that they are unable to go through with the act when partners are available. It does seem in this day and age that girls who remain virgins (unless they have strong backing in religious beliefs) are likely to worry about their normality. The questions I hear in discussion sessions indicate some shame over virginity. It is as though the virginal girl fears that in remaining chaste she fails to prepare herself for the responsibility of love and marriage.

The Problems of Boys

I have said little about the impact of changes in sexual attitudes upon the mental health of boys. From a moral standpoint there has been little concern about boys. Neither those who advocate liberalism nor those who favor a double standard worry much when boys have abundant opportunities for sex. Yet there are a few aspects of the new sexuality that seem to have an adverse effect upon male students.

One problem is again created by the mass communication media which suggests that sex is everywhere available. There are dozens of sources telling boys that girls are more promiscuous than ever. The boy who chooses to abstain or who has difficulty in finding a partner feels more freakish than ever. When boys do have an opportunity for sex they sometimes take a desperately exploitative attitude toward their partners. Some of the competitive aspects of the new sexuality are manifested in a mechanical striving for perfection. Our clinic sees an increasing number of unmarried men who complain of impotence, premature ejaculation, and inability to have an ejaculation. My impression is that male patients feel under more pressure than ever before to prove themselves through the sex act. Many experience difficulty simply because they are more interested in status than in the tender aspects of lovemaking.

Efforts to prove masculinity through multiple conquests are still common. Those boys who are able to become part of the promiscuous subculture find it convenient to pursue sex as a kind of aggressive game. Many male students are tempted to postpone commitment to one person. Instead they lead the kind of life advocated by the *Playboy* philosophy. In earlier years some of these men might have been seduced into marriage in order to gain sexual gratification. While this old-fashioned resolution was unhealthy for some, it may have been quite healthy for others. Today, a man who fears closeness to or intimacy with a woman has fewer opportunities to resolve his problems. The casualness of his sexual encounters precludes his desiring or becoming entrapped in a relationship which might have eventually resolved his fears of intimacy.

Conclusions

It is far too early to evaluate the psychological consequences of our sexual revolution. I would, however, like to make a few observations.

First, it seems clear that changes in sexual attitudes and practices do have an influence upon the mental health of some students. The nature of this influence however is too complex to allow for generalizations as to whether a given practice is either good or bad for people. Psychiatrists at one time impugned Victorian sexual attitudes and considered them an important cause of mental illness. They advocated more permissiveness and our society has moved toward more permissiveness. And what has happened? Our patient load has not decreased, yet the majority of our youthful patients are not repressed or inhibited people. Rather, today's patient is characterized by a high degree of sexual freedom and self-indulgence. The proposition that gratification of sexual needs is highly correlated with mental health seems to be at least questionable.

While I have pointed out the manner in which permissive sexual practices can potentiate mental illness, it would be equally dangerous to conclude that permissive sexual behavior is universally unhealthy. It may be true that our promiscuous patients are unhealthy, but there may be many promiscuous girls who never visit psychiatrists who are quite happy. The psychiatrist simply lacks information about the population as a whole. Until we know much more than we do now, we would be wise to stop generalizing about the relationship of sex to mental health.

At the same time that a psychiatrist must be wary of generalization, once he confronts a patient as an individual he does have some responsibility to help that person decide what is right or wrong. How does he do this? If we were to try to describe an ethical principle by which psychiatrists operate, we would have to include the psychiatrist's commitment to help the patient do what is best for himself, that is, to help the patient lead the most gratifying and most useful life without inflicting pain upon himself or others. Confronted with new sexual attitudes and practices which impose new stresses upon his patients, the psychiatrist finds that he often must interpose himself between a "thou shalt not" and an "anything goes" philosophy. He does this by repeatedly asking his patient, "Are you being honest with yourself? Will this behavior hurt you or those you love? Will it be good for you? Is it really what you want?"

A final consideration is whether psychiatrists or other physicians can help prevent mental illness which is associated with the sexual revolution. Certainly, providing sexual information which is not sensationalized, exaggerated, or contaminated by myth will help many young people make rational decisions about their future conduct. There may also be more specific preventive measures which discourage aimless and unsatisfying promiscuity.

A girl is most vulnerable to promiscuity shortly after she terminates a sexual relationship with her first lover. She has usually elected to give up her virginity because of a commitment to a boy she eventually hopes to marry. When she discovers that their relationship will not be permanent, she experiences a sense of depression over her loss and a sense of freedom from conventional restraints. Both factors militate toward promiscuous sexuality. It would be desirable for every young person who has just terminated an intense sexual relationship to have some opportunity for professional counseling. Perhaps an even more important need is to help our youth understand those conditions which favor and those conditions which interfere with a permanent relationship. If students were more capable of gauging the depth of commitment in their relationships, they would be in a better position to make the initial decisions as to their premarital sexual behavior.

OUR ROLE IN THE GENERATION, MODIFICATION, AND TERMINATION OF LIFE

Robert H. Williams, M.D.

My interests in certain philosophical aspects of medicine were accentuated by medical students who urged me to offer some elective courses in this sphere. These and many other experiences have prompted me to include coverage in my presidential address of such major and timely topics as population control, genetic bioengineering, abortion, transplantation, superbiological functions, suicide, and euthanasia. Handicaps to progress in these issues include ancient policies in religion, laws, and social philosophy. New drugs, life-sustaining apparatus, and organ replacements are provoking important moral, philosophical, psychological, social, economic, medical, and legal questions.

Population problems. Our biggest future concerns are hyperpopulation and its subquality. The population doubling time has decreased enormously, to thirty-seven years. Problems of clothing, food, jobs, housing, and other factors are multiplying rapidly. Unrest, murders, riots, violence, and wars will increase. It is estimated that 3,500,000 people, chiefly children, will die this year of starvation. Hardin states, "Freedom to breed will bring ruin to all." Others, however, maintain that all actions concerning the number and type of the population should be based upon voluntary decisions.

Questionnaire. In order to obtain opinions from a segment of leaders in American medicine I submitted a questionnaire to each member of the Association of Professors of Medicine, the Association of American Physicians, or both. A total of 344 responses was obtained, representing 97 percent of those questioned.

Generation of Life

Antifertility measures. Antifertility drugs taken orally have the widest field of application for population control, but, especially in the group needing them the most, numerous errors in the timing and dosages occur. Recently a medroxyprogesterone acetate preparation, injected quarterly, was reported to be 100 percent effective in preventing pregnancy, and its side effects were not prohibitive. The questionees were asked if they favored having the government provide such a compound free to all married women and to all single women over twenty-one years old who request it. Approximately 80 percent favored it for the married and single ones. About one-half favored offering a cash incentive with each injection to certain individuals with psychiatric, physical, social, or economic problems.

Abortion. Rather than such drugs, Japan has used abortion for reducing its birthrate to one of the lowest of any country in the world. Britain, Sweden, and other countries have liberalized their abortion laws to distinct advantage. Our enormously restrictive abortion laws cause extensive mental and physical suffering as well as major social, economic, and other problems. Our laws have not prevented abortion; about one million abortions are performed each year. Of those who have abortions, 10 percent are eventually hospitalized, and five thousand to ten thousand die. Of the abortions performed, 80 percent are performed on married women impregnated by their husbands. These women are chiefly thirty to forty years of age, with an average of two or more children. Some groups condone abortion when performed before "life begins" or before "the soul enters the body"; some select "quickening" as the time of soul entrance. As Lederberg has emphasized, life began many centuries ago. Quickening only symbolizes a very early phase of the recapitulation of phylogeny by ontogeny.

Experience shows that there is almost no mortality and very little morbidity from abortions performed by competent physicians in a licensed hospital. Eighty-six percent voted that the criminal abortion laws should be made inapplicable to licensed physicians and to women under the care of a physician. Almost all voted that such an abortion should be performed in an accredited hospital, and that physicians and others objecting to abortion should not be required to engage in it. The major bases for abortion should be the mental and physical status of the mother and child, and the effects on social, economic, and other conditions pertinent to the family and to society.

Amniocentesis. Amniocentesis is rapidly becoming a very important guide for selective abortions because important conditions are diagnosable by it, e.g., Down's syndrome, galactosemia, phenylketonuria, cystic fibrosis, and many others. At about the sixteenth week, amniotic fluid is withdrawn for chemical, histological, and other examinations, including cell cultures. There is relatively little morbidity and mortality. An abortion is desirable in some disorders. Other therapies may be instituted. With galactosemia, galactose is removed from the diet; for orotic aciduria, cytodylic and uridylic acids are given. In many instances, genetic counseling and other advisory approaches can be of great advantage. We may become active in changing genetic patterns.

Modification of Life

Euphenics. Euphenics, described by Lederberg as the "reprogramming of somatic cells and the modification of development," offers promise. Simple genetic messages can be synthesized chemically; genes can be prepared from one strain of bacteria and inserted into another, with the resulting cells and progeny programmed according to the messages and yielding respective responses (Nirenberg). Man may be able to program himself with synthetic information in the future. Experimental lines of special interest are the following: (1) viruses as carriers of genetic messages; (2) transplantation of cell nucleus; and (3) hybridization of cells from the same or different species. When nucleotide sequences are added to tobacco mosaic virus and the complex inoculated in tobacco plants, a systemic disease results indicating there has been a replication of the injected nucleotide complex. Other viruses have been used similarly. Since ribonucleic acid and deoxyribonucleic acid viruses have been replicated in vitro, possibly either after replication or de novo synthesis of certain nucleotides, the produce may be complexed with certain select viruses for introduction into a mammalian cell, leading to a reprogramming of the cell's activities. For example, the nucleic acid sequences bearing the code for phenylalanine hydroxylase synthesis might be attached to the virus and this complex could possibly be used as a vaccine for treating the phenylketonuria.

The nucleus of a fertilized egg might be replaced by the nucleus of a cultured cell and the resulting cell would have reprogrammed activity. It has been demonstrated that human cells which have been exposed to simian virus (SV 40) fused with mouse cells, and that the human-mouse cell hybrid, with its changed program, could be cultured for generations. While waiting for better cell generation, we are replenishing the old.

Organ transplantation. Surgeons have demonstrated good technical ability in transplanting heart and kidney. Even brain transplants in dogs have been active for a few days, but cerebral tissue establishes meaningful neuroanatomical association poorly. In the distant future, it might be possible to successfully transplant a head, thereby keeping the brain and the cranial nerves intact (White). When immunological and technological problems are solved, a sufficient number of organs cannot be supplied except by use of postmortem tissue. Some heart donors consist of those who have brain death before heart death. Criteria have been formulated to establish brain death, including deep and irreversible coma, the persistence of an isoelectric electroencephalogram, etc. The Uniform Anatomical Gift Act authorizes donation by individuals eighteen years of age or older *before* death, and donation by next of kin *after* death, of all or any part of the human body. This act has received enthusiastic approval by many groups, including 98 percent of the physicians I questioned. A proposal has been made by Dukeminier and Sanders for a law which would permit routine autopsy and organ removal for medical purposes unless the subject or next of kin has objected. This places the responsibility upon the patient and his next of kin to object rather than the physician having to seek permission routinely. The proposers emphasized that the plan would cause less mental trauma and give better results. Their proposal was favored by 71 percent of the questionees in my survey. Although the proposal has certain advantages, attempts for enaction should be delayed until as many states as possible adopt the Uniform Anatomical Gift Act and observe its effectiveness. Then decisions should be made concerning modifications and new measures.

In the future, one person might receive several organs, e.g., heart, liver, kidney, and possibly brain. The kidney is largely a filter, the heart chiefly a pump, and the liver a multiple servant, but the brain performs the major function of the body, *mentation*. All of the other organs are subservient to mentation. The brain recipient presumably would have aspects of mentation possessed by the donor, including origination of thoughts, perception, memory, and correlation, at least as far as they are influenced by the brain's inherent chemical reactions. Abnormal amounts and types of compounds released by nonbrain structures, which penetrate the blood-brain barrier, also influence mentation. Presumably, a normal brain transplanted successfully into a patient with phenylketonuria or Lesch-Nyhan syndrome, would experience significant alterations in mentation.

Mentation. Mentation and soul relations must be evaluated because we have been taught to visualize the soul as our supreme guide in moral issues, and all of the topics discussed herein have major moral aspects. It is difficult to visualize a soul in a hydrocephalic child or in one who has always been in coma. It seems unlikely that a person who never has any thoughts derives any meaning from the Bible or from sermons. In other words, what we visualize as a soul appears to be a specialized aspect of mentation.

The amount and type of mentation depends on the body's chemical or physical status or both; no psychiatric entities develop without abnormality in either status. Alterations in the chemical or physical state or both can be produced by genetic, nutritional, metabolic, drug, social, psychological, and numerous other environmental factors. Lesch-Nyhan syndrome is a good example of how one enzyme defect can lead to marked behavioral changes. This disease of males is an X-linked recessive disorder, characterized by hypoxanthineguanine phosphoribosyl transferase deficiency. Clinically, there are signs of mental retardation, and aggressive, compulsive, self-mutilative behavior, such as chewing of lips, gums, cheeks, and fingers. In most mental conditions, the specific primary etiology has not been elucidated, but an increasing number of chemical alterations are being correlated with them, e.g., as reported with phenylketonuria, homocystinuria, histidinemia, and hyperparathyroidism. Such chemical-behavioral interrelations should stimulate greater searches by us in our clinical experiences dealing with many "neurotics."

Termination of Life

Problems of the aged. Mental agony is high in the aged. This group is involved more than others in the problems of suicide and euthanasia. They are inappropriately handled in a large number of ways. Each medical school has a Department of Pediatrics, but probably less than 10 percent have an excellent Department or Division of Gerontology. We should throw away our congeries of rationalization and face extensively and soon this highly important problem.

We all know of certain individuals who have worked hard all of their lives, have amassed fame, fortune, and many honors, and have dreamed of millennium upon retirement: plenty of time for rich pleasures, recreation, and sweet memories of their glorious handiwork. Later years bring mental and physical tortures, feelings of marked loneliness and uselessness, and of being a burden to relatives, friends, and society. Others have had these later years of distress superimposed upon a lifetime of social, economic, mental, and physical problems. One with either pattern may look hopefully to the day when all of his troubles are gone, but have the dream shattered by therapies given by a physician who has only *one* consideration—to prolong life, no matter what else is involved. Our goal should *not* be to prolong every life as long as possible, with the use of all possible methods, including extensive use of drugs, operations, organ transplantation, artificial organs, respirators, hemodialyzers, cross-circulation, pacemakers, etc., irrespective of whether such prolongation leads to happiness, or to great physical and/or mental suffering in the patient and others.

Suicide. With this setting there is no wonder that the suicide rate rises with aging of men. Although the Bible does not specifically condemn suicide some religions regard it as the "most fatal of sins." Certain laws label it a felony. The victims are visualized by some members of society as cowards and weaklings; strong stigmata prevail for them and their families. With so many punitive implications, castigations, and marked lack of understanding and sympathy, many potential suicide victims contend alone with their problems, at least until they have attained a severe state of depression, anxiety, agitation, frustration, and other agony. Because of their great distress and exhaustion, many cannot analyze their problems satisfactorily and commit suicide in desperation. The extent of their suffering is emphasized by the horrible means of death selected by some. However, the greatest horror in these cases usually is not death but the torture which preceded it. It is easy for those who are not undergoing the same agony to advocate calmness and clear thinking, but this often is analogous to telling a person who is sitting on a red-hot burner to sit calmly and remain cool. If all elements of society had a better approach to suicide, the potential victims would seek aid sooner and be treated more effectively.

If enormous agonies persist after expert attention to potential suicide victims for appropriate periods of time, should euthanasia be considered? Euthanasia, with appropriate approval, seems more desirable than suicide. Since we make great efforts to keep a patient alive when he desires it, should we give more attention to his wishes when he desires euthanasia? Some victims have weighed carefully the pros and cons and have decided that what *they* will gain and contribute to others by continuing to live does not justify their tremendous mental and physical agony. Sometimes the decision is wise. Some of them would endure these agonies if they felt that their survival would significantly benefit others, themselves, or both.

Euthanasia. Euthanasia has been used for many purposes since early history. The questionees were asked: with appropriate change in laws, detailed consideration of the status of the patient and others by this physician and two or more additional professional hospital personnel, and with consent of the patient or appropriate relative or both, do you favor in certain carefully selected instances (a) negative euthanasia (planned omission of therapies that would prolong life) or (b) positive euthanasia (institution of therapy that is hoped will promote death sooner than otherwise)? Eighty-seven percent favored negative euthanasia, and 15 percent favored positive euthanasia; 80 percent signified that they had practiced negative euthanasia.

Negative euthanasia. Negative euthanasia has been applied much too infrequently, even though physicians and members of the public favor it in certain instances. Patients, their families, and friends experience far more physical and mental suffering than should occur. Some patients lead a vegetative existence for months or years; heart-lung perfusion and other subsidiary functions continue, but the prime function, mentation, has gone. Such customs are continued chiefly because of certain religious policies, laws, and fears of death. More effort should be made to reduce fears of death itself; I have gone almost entirely through the "pearly gates" and did not find it so bad.

The Almighty set up the genetic pattern to assure death. The Bible states that there is a "time to die." Reverend Sullivan says that "suffering is almost the greatest gift of God's love." Extending such reasoning, we might ask them why should we interfere with the progress of diseases that may lead to death? Why should we use anesthesia for operations, or, indeed, why should we even operate? Pope Pius XII stated that in a deeply unconscious, hopeless case, there should not be an attempt to continue to maintain the bodily functions by extraordinary means. Some have stated that legal approval of euthanasia would "weaken our moral fiber." However, I believe that our moral fiber must be weak to permit certain instances of prolonged marked suffering.

Positive euthanasia. A major deterrent to positive euthanasia has been: "Thou shalt not kill." However, Leviticus says, "He who kills a man shall be put to death" (Lev. 24:17), and Ecclesiastes states there is "a time to be born, and a time to die . . . a time to kill, and a time to heal" (Eccles. 3:2a,3). We recognize justifiable homicide in self-defense, in capital punishment, and in extensive wars. We hold guiltless "murderers of unsound mind." Terminating life seems justified with abortion, sterilization, and spermicidal agents. Is it not justifiable in certain situations which will cause tremendous mental and physical suffering and other problems to a given patient, his relatives, friends, and society?

In certain patients, a very remote possibility of recovery does not seem sufficient counterjustification. Some individuals favor positive euthanasia but fear its abuse and the difficulties of making decisions in various situations.

Comment

We must be patient and make progress step by step in the right direction. Although we have been proceeding extremely slowly, we must also be cautious about progressing too rapidly. There should be appropriate changes in laws and policies after extensive consideration by many different segments of society: physicians, religious leaders, legislators, sociologists, psychologists, and others. We should formulate procedures that would be best for society, while protecting certain rights and desires of individuals and groups. Although it would be best to establish uniform policies, we will probably not get support from all religious groups, because they have different philosophies. It would be best not to force these groups to conform unless nonconformity would affect society or significant segments of it too adversely. We should have appropriate committees and consultants to deal with special problems that arise.

Finally, I wish to emphasize that the topics discussed are ones that trigger strong emotional reactions—indeed, ones that often stifle good reason and progress. Present policies prompt many unnecessary mental, physical, social, economic, and other problems. Institution of major changes will necessitate hard work by many people. We of the noble profession of medicine should *lead* in proceeding as fast as wise planning, education, and general support permit. It is hoped that we will increase our activities *immediately* in population control, selective abortions, problems of mentation, aging, suicide, and negative euthanasia. Presently, it appears that longer intervals may be required for major application of genetic bioengineering, organ transplantation, and positive euthanasia. Whereas many of our goals will be temporarily thwarted, I hope we will have the courage, determination, and dedication to attain them.

EXTREME MEASURES TO PROLONG LIFE

One of the clinical dilemmas I have encountered concerns the care of the terminally ill patient. Not infrequently life can be prolonged only by extraordinary therapeutic measures. Is it the physician's duty to preserve a patient's life simply because it is scientifically possible to do so? I do not refer to use of a drug or other treatment to hasten death but rather to withholding strenuous and possibly costly therapy in instances of incurable disease. Should the professed wish of the relatives play a dominant role in this situation?

RESPONDENT: *Very Rev. Brian Whitlow, D.D.*

The problem we are concerned with is one which arises not from medical failure but from unparalleled medical success. When we consider its moral implications, we must beware of placing too much reliance on traditional morality. This may prove an uncertain guide to us who are faced with cases of a kind unknown when the traditions were formed. We ought rather to look for the basic moral principles from which in our time particular guidelines may be adduced for the new situation.

Let me begin by offering some unconnected observations. Then I will attempt a conclusion.

There is no obligation to preserve a patient's life merely because it is medically possible to do so.

A certain sentimentality sometimes enters into the problem. When deep unconsciousness has descended, the patient, as far as can be known, is not suffering at all. An argument for shortening his life based on pity for his suffering is therefore misconceived. It is his relatives and those who care for him who suffer, because they see him in a pitiable condition. They feel this acutely and project their feelings onto the patient.

The wish of the patient (if it could be known from previously expressed opinion) would be relevant, but only to a limited degree. If the withholding of care or drug is wrong (either in law or morals), it is still wrong even though the patient may be presumed to have given his consent.

Nor can the wishes of relatives be taken as providing an ultimate sanction. The physician is not a veterinarian. A veterinarian's patient is the animal, but his client is the animal's owner; the decision, whether the animal lives or dies, lies legally and morally with the owner. But the physician's responsibility to his patient is personal and primary. He cannot allow himself to become the agent of the patient's relatives. They may have a sinister interest in his death, or a pecuniary interest in his staying alive until a certain date.

Therefore, society should not take the duty of decision away from the doctor, though the burden of moral decision should not be his exclusively. Perhaps for fear of malpractice suits, some physicians continue with extreme protestations of loyalty to the final spark of life, unqualified by the patient's ability to continue living as a person.

The physician should not have to bear the burden alone. But he must remain answerable for his decision to society and to God. He himself may have other interests in his patient. He may have expectations under the patient's will; he may have legitimate interests in medical research. We live in a time of widening exploration of new surgical and other techniques. Society requires adequate safeguards that such scientific experimentation remains subordinate to the interests of the patient as a person.

There must inevitably be a period of uncertainty until medical clarification of the new situation results in a new legal definition of death. Law does not create nor dictate morality but is one custodian of it. If the irretrievably unconscious person is "alive," he enjoys all the protection which the law affords to a living person.

Some Theological Observations

I believe that our problem arises not only from successful modern ingenuities which have brought certain moral complications to the process of dying, but also from a changed philosophical climate in society as a whole. Many of our North American ethical codes and moral presuppositions are derived from the Christian religion in which a large section of society no longer believes. We live in an increasingly post-Christian age. The effect of this is noticeable in the matter with which we are concerned here. A growing agnosticism has made people uncertain about life after death. This has given to the moment of death a finality which it did not have previously.

The notion in much contemporary thought, that life as such (the vital or biological principle) is the highest good, is an error. It is far removed from the Christian view that there are many things more important than mere existence.

The Christian does not respect life any less for recognizing the boon of death. Because life is what it is, there frequently comes a moment when it is good to die (and therefore good to allow another to go unvexed to death). Where Christian insight is deepest, death itself, when it comes, has an element in it of voluntary surrender. Christ himself died with the words "Father, into thy hands I commend my spirit," (Luke 23:46, K.J.V.) and history records many examples of others who have passed into the experience of death in the same way.

If the Christian physician concludes that death, not recovery, is God's will for the patient, he will believe himself morally justified in ceasing to obstruct the process of dying and in beginning instead to cooperate with it.

Traditional Christian moralists draw a distinction between "ordinary" and "extraordinary" medical or surgical procedures. This view was well restated recently by Pope Pius XII in an allocution to physicians in November 1957.

By "ordinary" in this sense, the theologian does not mean

what the physician would regard as normal treatment. It means whatever treatment a patient can obtain and undergo without imposing an excessive burden on himself or others. A sick man is bound (as are those who have the care of him) to employ the available means of preserving life and restoring health.

"Extraordinary" treatment has been defined as "what is very costly, or very painful, or very difficult, or very dangerous." A patient is not bound to submit to extraordinary treatment (so defined) unless he has some special obligation to stay alive. Nor is the doctor bound to apply such extraordinary treatment in cases where the patient cannot be consulted.

The fairly clear traditional distinction in Christian casuistry does not exactly fit our dilemma but may be helpful in some cases.

I would add that many of the mechanical procedures now in use ought perhaps to be regarded in their proper nature as temporary. Their normal function is to win time for the restorative measures to take effect. If, after they have been given a fair trial according to the circumstances of the case, it becomes evident that the patient can never be restored to functioning on his own, it may be said that the mechanical procedures have failed in their purpose. All they are doing is keeping the patient in a condition of artificially arrested death, and they should therefore be discontinued.

A Tentative Conclusion

I mentioned the difficulties which result from our pluralistic society in which dying patients and those who attend them may include devout Christians, convinced atheists, uncertain agnostics, and everything in between.

For the priest (I include, of course, all ministers of religion in this term), much depends upon the religious suppositions shared between him and the patient. He may know the patient to have been a person who, in the days of his health, loved God and was obedient to that love. The patient may have prepared himself over the years for death. In such cases, the priest would not be troubled by the desire to prolong technical life for a few extra weeks, by the exact moment of legal death, or by whether the patient could ever be brought back to consciousness.

The difficulties arise when he is called to help people who do not accept or understand the Christian view of death. This may include the physician. In such cases, the priest must fall back upon the general observations with which I began, and which do in fact provide certain guidelines.

In my view, essential medical or nursing care must always be given: food, warmth, washing, and easing of bodily position. But beyond that, decisions must be left to the physician. Medical opinion must always be the basis for deciding whether there is any reasonable hope of recovery.

An underlying principle of Christianity is that the love of God and of one's neighbors must be given priority at all times. Christ respected the Ten Commandments and the other traditional laws but gave this principle a priority over them all. I believe that the Christian position in the end comes to this: if the doctor is sincerely and selflessly trying to do the best for his patient, he is more likely to take the right course than if we try to draw up hard-and-fast rules to guide him in all cases.

RESPONDENT: *Fred Rosner, M.D.*

The problem raised exemplifies what may be called passive medical intervention in relation to termination of a patient's life, that is, the situation in which therapy is withheld so that death is hastened by omission of treatment. Active medical intervention is the case when a drug or other treatment is administered, and death is thereby hastened. Both forms of medical intervention may be voluntary or involuntary, that is, with or without the patient's consent.

Religious attitudes toward such medical intervention in relation to termination of a patient's life are of prime importance in evaluating an individual case. The Roman Catholic Church states: ". . . the teaching of the Church is unequivocal that God is the supreme master of life and death and that no human being is allowed to usurp His dominion so as deliberately to put an end to life, either his own or anyone else's with authorization. . . . and the only authorizations the Church recognizes are a nation engaged in war, execution of criminals by a Government, killing in self defense. . . . The Church has never allowed and never will allow the killing of individuals on grounds of private expediency; for instance . . . putting an end to prolonged suffering or hopeless sickness. . . ." [1]

Thus we see a blanket condemnation by the Catholic Church as a mortal sin of active intervention in relation to termination of a patient's life. The reasons behind this teaching include the inviolability of human life or the supreme domination of God over his creatures and the purposefulness of human suffering. Man suffers as penance for his sins. Passive medical intervention, however, has been sanctioned by Pope Pius XII, who issued an encyclical in the last year of his life not requiring a physician to use "extraordinary" measures when certain death and suffering lie ahead. In this age of auxiliary hearts, artificial kidneys, respirators, pacemakers, defibrillators, and similar instruments, the definition of "extraordinary" is unclear and nebulous, however.

In the Protestant churches there exist "all possible colors in the spectrum of attitudes" [2] toward medical intervention in relation to termination of a patient's life. Some condemn it, some favor it, and many are in between, advocating judgment of each case individually.

The Jewish attitude toward medical intervention in relation to terminating life is summarized by Jacobovits: ". . . any form of *active* [intervention] is strictly prohibited and condemned as plain murder. . . . anyone who kills a dying person is liable to the death penalty as a common murderer. At the same time, Jewish law sanctions . . . the withdrawal of any factor—whether extraneous to the patient himself or not—which may artificially delay his demise in the final phase." [3] Jacobovits is quick to point out, however, that all the Jewish sources refer to an individual in whom death is expected to be imminent (three days or less in rabbinic references). Thus, passive medical intervention in a patient who may yet live for weeks or months may not necessarily be condoned.

The moral, ethical, legal, and religious arguments for and against medical intervention in relation to terminating a patient's life are numerous, and there are lengthy discussions on the subject.[4] The physician is in a predicament: on the one hand, it is his duty to relieve suffering, yet, on the other hand, he must preserve and protect life. The problem is well stated: "When a tortured man asks, 'For God's sake doctor, let me die, just put me to sleep,' we have yet to find the answer as to whether to comply *is* for God's sake, the patient's sake, our own or possibly all three."[5]

Even if the moral and religious questions could be circumvented, problems of logistics would immediately arise. Who is to initiate the proceedings for medical intervention? the patient? the family? the physician? a group of physicians? the courts? Who is to carry out the decision if it is affirmative? the physicians? others?

In conclusion, there is no general answer available to the question of medical intervention in relation to termination of a patient's life. Each case must be individualized. Most people would probably agree that withholding of treatment or discontinuation of instrumentation and machinery in an incurably ill patient would be permitted if one were certain that in doing so he is shortening the act of dying and not interrupting life. Yet who can make the fine distinction between prolonging life and prolonging the act of dying? The former comes within the physician's reference; the latter does not.

PROLONGATION OF LIFE OR PROLONGING THE ACT OF DYING?

One of my patients has advanced cerebral arteriosclerosis and had been in a state of semiconsciousness for three months. The nutrition of this aged woman is maintained by means of stomach-tube feeding and occasional parenteral feedings. This is obviously an incurable disease, and the patient would not recognize family members even if she were to become somewhat more alert. In comparable instances, such as in patients with incurable diseases which are very painful, or when maintenance of life in the incurable patient results in great financial hardship, does the physician have the obligation or right to prolong life under all circumstances? Who decides?

RESPONDENT: *William P. Williamson, M.D.*

In this particular instance, it could aptly be said that the tube feedings and parenteral administrations are prolonging dying, not living. A physician has a responsibility to ease suffering in those hopeless situations where there is no medical doubt as to the outcome. This patient is incompetent to enter into any decision about her medical management, so decisions here must be made between physicians and the family, and hopefully, with the appropriate clergyman in consultation on the matter. If there is full agreement with the family, if the involved clergyman concurs, and if decision is reached after careful discussion at a high level of integrity involving medical judgment, emotions of the family, ethics, and religion, then I feel such artificial feedings may be discontinued. Routine daily feedings by mouth can be offered, and if this particular patient is not able to partake, then I see no moral, legal, or spiritual obligation to institute tube feedings, which in this instance can be regarded as "extraordinary," heroic, or not medically indicated. This feeding is not designed to build up her physical condition to face some attempt at curative medical or surgical therapy. It is a senseless, deliberate prolongation of suffering and dying. However, unless all can agree on this course of action, including family, clergyman, and physician, then one must carry on with these artificial measures of nourishment.

The physician should treat the patient within the dictates of the patient's religion and philosophy, and not try to force his own moral, philosophical, or religious decisions on others. The physician may withdraw from the case if his own religious or moral beliefs produce a conflict which he cannot conscientiously handle.

In comparable instances, each patient and situation must be assessed individually. Because of countless variables, rigid rules are not only impossible but they are also unjustified. One should not practice medicine by rule, but by reason. Communication is the answer—free, honest, open, and intelligent, between patient, family, physician, and clergyman.

In questionable cases, I agree with Laforet, who stated that "to err on the side of active treatment" is wiser than laissez-faire, for the following reasons:

> 1. The physician is fallible, and the case may *not* be medically "hopeless." 2. The physician by tradition has been committed to *active* contention with disease. 3. The physician is not competent to determine fully the "quality" of a given life or whether longevity is "fruitless." 4. Even if without positive act, the physician who arrogates to himself the prerogative of determining whether life shall continue or terminate by default is in an uncomfortable moral position. 5. The discovery of new curative agents is an ever present possibility. 6. Spontaneous regression of malignancies in apparently "hopeless" patients has been documented. 7. Miraculous intervention is possible. 8. The physician may find that self-recrimination at errors of omission is harsher than at errors of commission. 9. Even a brief moment of mental lucidity in a mori-

bund patient may be all-important for his spiritual welfare. 10. "Extraordinary" means of treatment may result in cure.[1]

However, in the stated case, there appears to be no possible chance of return to any type of conscious awareness, much less any comfortable existence. To me, this act of omitting tube feedings in this patient in this circumstance is not euthanasia in subterfuge; it is good medicine.

RESPONDENT: *Fred W. Reid, Jr., Chaplain*

In the wake of modern medicine's tremendous advances in technology I wonder if we do not find ourselves in danger of our science outrunning our art. We have moved swiftly from the role of the doctor in the horse and buggy who was the physician, counselor, and financial adviser to the hypertrained physician who in his practice of medicine concerns himself with monitoring units, organ transplants, and other technological devices capable of prolonging the patient's life. With such instruments and knowledge, the physician is frequently faced with such decisions as the one presented in this question dealing with the patient who has advanced cerebral arteriosclerosis and has been in this state of semiconsciousness for a three-month period.

The main issue at stake seems to be whether the physician is actually prolonging this patient's life or whether by this thera-peutic treatment he is preventing the patient's death. Such decisions on the part of the physician embrace many more con-cerns than just whether the patient's electrolytes are in balance or what constitutes the blood chemistry. These judgments have moral and ethical implications which take into consideration the patient as a whole man. As the physician attempts to deal with this patient in a holistic framework, he immediately finds himself involved with a team approach in medicine. Many times the family in consultation with the physician can be extremely ben-eficial in helping the physician see the total implications of this patient's life. If this patient has a meaningful relationship with a religious faith, then the clergyman of that faith can be of assistance to the physician on the moral and ethical implications of the decisions being made. In this way the physician is not treating the disease alone but is treating the patient as a whole person.

Increasingly this kind of terminally ill situation presents itself in our medical centers today. We do possess the knowledge and ability to prolong life and prevent death. Someone has to make the medical, moral, and ethical decision as to which is the case in a given situation. Thus it is by no coincidence that moral and ethical issues are on the frontier of medicine today. Many of our medical schools throughout the country are addressing themselves to these kinds of issues in an effort to prepare the physician to deal more effectively with these difficult situations. Perhaps one of the modifications that should and, I feel, will occur is the way in which the law looks at this particular aspect of medicine. According to Edwin J. Holman: "The law should reflect what is moral, what is right and what is wrong. The law does not and should not determine what is moral. In areas of morality the law should not express a position concerning the rightness or wrongness of conduct in the absence of sound moral discussion and agreement." [2] This statement would appear to place the burden of responsibility in determining what is moral upon the church, our educational institutions, and upon us as members of this society in which we live. Therefore, this presents an even stronger challenge to face up to what moral and ethical issues are involved in medicine today and to deal with them as comprehensively as possible. One way that is open to the physician is the above-mentioned team approach which involves the family, the minister, and the physician as they together attempt to decide what is best for the patient.

Today the church is under pressing obligation to address itself to these difficult areas with which the doctor is daily having to struggle. Many of our religious groups are already in the process of beginning to take a hard look at such moral and ethical considerations as extraordinary measures for prolonging life, along with other implications of modern medical technology. This action in itself can further constitute a resource for the physician as he attempts to treat the patient as a whole person.

LEGAL ASPECTS OF THE DECISION NOT TO PROLONG LIFE

George P. Fletcher, J.D.

New medical techniques for prolonging life force the legal and medical professions to reexamine their traditional attitudes toward life and death. The new set of problems emerges from the following recurrent situation: a comatose patient has a flat electroencephalogram reading; according to the best judgment, he has an infinitesimal chance of recovery; he can be sustained by intravenous therapy. What should his physician do? In making his decision, how much weight should the physician give to the wishes of the family, to the financial condition of the family, and to the prospect that his time might be profitably used in caring for patients with a better chance for recovery?

It would be a mistake to think that our legal tradition contains clear answers to these questions. If this type of case demands moral sensitivity of the physician, it demands much more of the legal theorist and of the legislator. For, in confronting this type of case, the legal theorist must be concerned not only with situations in which the physician in the case is bestowed with sensitivity to the moral issues, but also with cases in which the physician and the family involved might be moved by lesser motives. The lawyer must be concerned about formulating legal norms that would permit a just resolution of the "clear" cases without providing an opportunity for abuse.

If one were to have a legal standard endorsing the physician's decision not to prolong life, should the standard be limited to the case of a doomed comatose patient with a flat EEG reading? Consider how this case blends so gradually into many related cases. First, there is the case of the doomed comatose patient who still shows some signs of brain activity. Does this patient *deserve* prolongation of life? Neither he nor his brother with a flat EEG reading can enjoy the beauties of life on earth. Why should we keep him alive? Second, compare the case of the doomed but conscious patient who can perceive the world about him but who suffers excruciating pain. Is the fact of consciousness and the fact of an EEG reading sufficient to say that this man must be kept alive? In analyzing the physician's legal obligation to prolong a patient's life, we should keep in mind the infinitely graduated spectrum from the clear cases to the cases that are far from clear. The essential difficulty is formulating standards for separating cases on one end of the spectrum from those on the other end.

There are a number of significant topics in the laws' relationship to the problem of prolonging life and to the more general problem of euthanasia. In recent years, we have seen a number of efforts toward legalizing voluntary euthanasia, i.e., cases in which the patient is said to have consented to the termination of his life. Literature abounds with vigorous debate for and against these proposals; Williams and Kamisar present current debate on the subject.[1] A general survey of this related problem may also be found in the literature.[2] Yet the term "prolongation of life" conveys a slightly different meaning from that suggested by the term "euthanasia." The first term carries a suggestion of artificially lengthening a life that would otherwise end. In contrast, the latter term, "euthanasia," sometimes called "mercy killing," suggests a beneficent termination of life that might otherwise continue. In speaking about voluntary euthanasia in particular, one has in mind cases in which the good of ending a man's suffering allegedly outweighs the wrong of intentionally terminating a life. The subject of euthanasia has received considerable comment in the legal literature. Thus, in this paper, I shall limit my remarks to the special problems posed by the term "prolongation of life."

Acts and Omissions

One might begin legal analysis by considering one of the fundamental distinctions that runs through the law of crimes and of torts. This is the distinction between the acts and omissions, a distinction that has had a rich philosophical history as well. In acting, one intercedes to terminate life; one shoots and kills a man or one injects air into his veins. In omitting to act, one fails to intercede in order to preserve life and, as a result, permits death to occur. It is the difference between active and passive behavior. It is also the difference between causing harm and permitting harm to occur. It is indisputably clear in the law that acting to terminate life is first-degree murder. This is true regardless of the motives of the actor. At one time in the evolution of the common law of murder, it might have made a difference whether a man was moved by emotions of spite or by emotions of mercy. One speaks of the element of "malice" in the common law definition of murder. Surely a man does not kill maliciously if he kills in order to save another man from unbearable suffering. But the concept of "malice" lost its force in the evolution of the common law; as early as the sixteenth and seventeenth centuries it came to mean nothing more significant than the requirement that the killing be intentional. Since a man killing for reasons of mercy does indeed kill intentionally, he kills maliciously—at least, according to the special dictionary of the law.

Killing for reasons of mercy, like killing in order to rob one's victim, is murder. But one should recognize that this statement of the law is a statement of principle only. There is a gap between the law in theory and the law in practice. That the legal norm is severe and uncompromising does not mean that the people who administer the legal system are also severe and uncompromising. Prosecutors or grand juries may fail to indict someone who is clearly guilty on the facts (and the acquittal is not appealable to a higher court); even after conviction, judges often suspend the sentences of men who killed to end the suffering of their victim.

A thorough discussion of particular cases reported in the press and the law reports is given by Kasimar.[3] Despite these institutional checks against the severity of the law, some men guilty of killing for reasons of mercy are convicted and punished by imprisonment. But these cases of actual conviction and punishment do not include beneficent killings by medical practitioners. There is no case in the Anglo-American tradition in which a doctor has been convicted of murder or manslaughter for having killed to end the suffering of his patient.[4]

The distinction between the law in theory and the law in action is critical when one turns to an examination of criminal or tort liability for omitting to render therapy and thus permitting a man to die. In this area, one can find no decided cases at all to support the theory of liability. Neither laymen nor doctors have been convicted of omitting to take steps that could have averted death. Yet it is clear as a matter of legal principle that a doctor would be liable for failing to take steps to save the life of his patient. One need only consider the following bizarre case. Dr. Brown is the family doctor of the Smith family and has been for several years. Tim Smith falls ill with pneumonia. Dr. Brown sees him once or twice at the family home and administers the necessary therapy. One evening, upon receiving a telephone call from the Smith family that Tim is in a critical condition, Dr. Brown decides that he should prefer to remain at his bridge game rather than to visit the sick Smith child. In this case, Brown fails to render aid to the child. It is unquestionably clear that Brown would be liable criminally and civilly if death should ensue. That he has merely omitted to act, rather than asserted himself intentionally to end life, makes no difference in assessing his criminal and civil liability.

Of course, the doctor would not be under an obligation to respond to the call of a stranger who said that he needed help. But there is a difference between a stranger and someone who has put himself in the care of a physician. The factor of reliance and reasonable expectation that the doctor will render aid means that the doctor is legally obligated to do so. His failure to do so is then tantamount to an intentional infliction of harm. And as his motive, be it for good or ill, is irrelevant in analyzing his liability for intentional and assertive killing, his motive is also irrelevant in analyzing his liability for omitting to render aid when he is obligated to do so. Thus, it makes no difference because he prefers to continue playing bridge or if he does so in the hope that the patient's misery will come quickly to a natural end.

Thus, a doctor may be criminally and civilly liable either for intentionally taking life or for omitting to act and thus permitting death to occur. But the sources of these two legal prescriptions are different. And this difference in the source of the law may provide the key for the analysis of the doctor's liability in failing to prolong life in the cases discussed at the outset of this article. That a doctor may not actively kill is an application of the general principle that no man may actively kill a fellow human being. In contrast, the principle that a doctor may not omit to render aid to a patient justifiably relying upon him is a function of the special relationship that exists between doctor and patient. In cases of actions resulting in death, the doctor's duty arises from the simple fact that he and his patients are human beings. In cases of omissions resulting in death, the doctor's duty arises from the relationship between him and his patient. Thus, in analyzing the doctor's legal duty to his patient, one must take into consideration whether the question involved is an act or an omission. If it is an act, the relationship between the doctor and patient is irrelevant. If it is an omission, the relationship is all-controlling.

Applying the Distinction

With these theoretical distinctions in mind, we may turn to an analysis of specific aspects of medical decision not to prolong life. The first problem is to isolate the relevant medical activity. The recurrent pattern includes stopping cardiac resuscitation, turning off the respirator, removing the needle used in intravenous therapy. The problem, of course, is whether these activities are to be regarded as cases of acts terminating life or of omissions to render aid to sustain life. For, as we have seen, this initial decision of classification determines the subsequent legal analysis of the case. If turning off the respirator is an "act" under the law, then it is unequivocally forbidden: it is on a par with injecting air into the patient's veins. If, on the other hand, it is classified as an "omission," the analysis proceeds more flexibly. Whether it would be forbidden as an omission would depend on the demands imposed by the relationship between doctor and patient.

There are gaps in the law, and we are confronted with one of them. There is simply no way to bring to bear the legal authorities to determine whether the process of turning off the respirator is an act or an omission. It looks very much like an act, for it takes physical movement to turn off the respirator. But that fact need not be controlling. There might be "acts" without physical movement, as, for example, if one should sit motionless in the driver's seat as one's car heads toward an intended victim. That would surely be an act causing death; it would be first-degree murder regardless of the relationship between the victim and his assassin. Similarly, there might be cases of omissions involving physical exertions, perhaps even the effort required to turn off the respirator. The problem is not whether there is or there is not physical movement; there must be another test.

That other test, I should propose, is whether on all the facts we should be inclined to speak of the activity as one that causes harm or one merely that permits harm to occur. The usage of the verbs "causing" and "permitting" corresponds to the distinction in the clear cases between acts and omissions. If one injects air into the veins of a doomed patient, he is causing harm. On the other hand, if the doctor fails to stop on the highway to aid a stranger injured in an automobile accident, it is difficult to say that the doctor is causing harm; he surely is permitting harm to occur, and he might be morally blameworthy for that; but as the verb "cause" is ordinarily used, his failing to stop is not the cause of the harm.

As native speakers of English, we are equipped with a linguistic sensitivity for the distinction between causing harm and permitting harm to occur. And we should employ that sensitivity in classifying the hard cases arising in discussions of the prolongation of life. Is turning off the respirator an instance of causing death or permitting death to occur? If the patient is beyond recovery and on the verge of death, one balks at saying that the activity causes death. It is far more natural to speak of the case as one of permitting death to occur. It is significant that we are inclined to refer to the respirator as a means for prolonging life; we wouldn't speak of treatment for pneumonia in the same way. The use of the term "prolongation of life" builds on the same perception of reality that prompts us to say that turning off the respirator is an activity permitting death to occur, rather than causing death. And that basic perception is that using the respirator interferes artificially in the pattern of events. Of course, the perception of the natural and of the artificial is a function of time and culture. What may seem artificial today may be a matter of course in ten years. Nonetheless, one *does* perceive many uses of the respirator today as artificial prolongations of life. And that sense of artificiality should be enough to determine the legal classification of the case. Because we are prompted to refer to the activity of turning off the respirator as activity permitting death to occur, rather than causing death, we may classify the case as an omission rather than as an act.

Let it be clear that using the label "omission" does not mean that the physician is free to do what he chooses, for he may be liable for omitting to do that which he is legally obligated to do. But moving from the arena of acts to the arena of omissions does yield some flexibility. Not all omissions are illegal; the problem is to determine which are and which are not. As we noted above, the legality of an omission to render aid depends on the relationship between the doctor and his patient. To take a clear case, let us suppose that prior to the onset of a terminal illness, the patient demands that his physician do everything to keep him alive and breathing as long as possible. And the physician responds, "Even if you have a flat EEG reading and there is no chance of recovery?" "Yes," the patient replies. If the doctor agrees to this bizarre demand, he does become obligated to keep the respirator going indefinitely. Thankfully, cases of this type do not occur in day-to-day medical practice. In the average case, the patient hasn't given a thought to the problem, and his physician is not likely to alert him to it. The problem then is whether there is an implicit understanding between physician and patient as to how the physician should proceed in the last stages of a terminal illness. An implicit understanding would be something akin to the expectation of a passenger on a bus that the driver plans to stop at the regular stops along the route. Might there be an understanding of that sort about what the physician should do if the patient is in a coma and dependent on a mechanical respirator? This is not the kind of thing regarding which the average man has expectations. And if he did, they would be expectations that would be based on the customary practices of the time. If he had heard about a number of cases in which patients had been sustained for long periods of time on respirators, he might (at least prior to going into the coma) expect that he would be similarly sustained.

Thus, the analysis leads us along the following path. The doctor's duty to prolong life is a function of his relationship with his patient, and, in the typical case, that relationship devolves into the patient's expectations of the treatment he will receive. Those expectations, in turn, are a function of the practices prevailing in the community at the time. And on what do those practices depend? Practices in the use of respirators to prolong life are no more and no less than what doctors actually do in the time and place. Thus, we have come full circle. We began the inquiry by asking: is it legally permissible for doctors to turn off respirators used to prolong the life of doomed patients? The answer after our tortuous journey is simply this: it all depends on what doctors customarily do. The law is sometimes no more precise than that.

The moral of our circular journey is that doctors are in a position to fashion their own law to deal with cases of prolongation of life. By establishing customary standards, they may determine the expectations of their patients and thus regulate the understanding and the relationship between doctor and patient. And by regulating that relationship, they may control their legal obligations to render aid to doomed patients.

Thus the medical profession confronts the challenge of developing humane and sensitive customary standards for guiding decisions to prolong the lives of terminal patients. This is not a challenge that the profession may shirk. For the doctor's legal duties to render aid derive from his relationship with the patient. That relationship, along with the expectations implicit in it, is the responsibility of the individual doctor and the individual patient. With respect to problems not commonly discussed by the doctor with his patient, particularly the problems of prolonging life, the responsibility for the patient's expectations lies with the medical profession as a whole.

It will not do for the medical profession to demand that we lawyers devise a legal definition of death. There might be many uses of a legal definition of death; one might wish to know the time of death to apply rules on the disposition of the decedent's estate. But this is not what medical practitioners have in mind. It seems that they should like to have a clear standard for deciding when and when not to render aid to their dying patients. Sweden's Dr. Crafoord has proposed that a patient be declared legally dead when his EEG reading is flat. The standard is clear and easy to apply, but it is morally insensitive. Should one totally disregard all the other factors: the likelihood of recovery, the family's financial position, the patient's expressed wishes, other demands on hospital facilities, and the attending physician's time? Even if we could formulate a just resolution of these conflicting factors today, would it be a resolution that would remain fair in the face of medical innovation? It surely would not. What one regards as excessive and extraordinary today might well become commonplace in a few years. A legal standard of death, which would define the limits of the doctor's duty to his patient, would be an overly rigid solution to a problem that changes dimensions with each medical innovation.

MANAGEMENT OF THE PATIENT WITH TERMINAL ILLNESS

Paul S. Rhoads, M.D.

When the physician is caring for a patient with a terminal illness, his duties go beyond doing everything that may reasonably be done to prolong life and relieve physical suffering. He has the obligation to tell the family, and usually the patient, the clinical facts and prognosis as truthfully as he knows them. Honesty often should be tempered with optimistic uncertainty. The physician must be in charge, refusing to listen to hindsight recriminations directed against colleagues, the patient, the patient's family, or himself after the final diagnosis has been made. With the patient's permission, he should enlist the help of the clergyman, if this has not already been done, and with him provide the spiritual support which the situation so urgently requires. How well he is able to do this will depend upon how well he, himself, has thought through the deeper problems of life and death.

The problems of incurable and life-threatening illness get right to the heart of the question of why we are physicians at all, and demand some soul-searching that goes beyond the facts and tools of our profession. They demand that we stop and do some hard thinking about ourselves, for the majority of us will, in the not too distant future, face the same fate as that of the patients we are trying to help. Will our final illness be a hopeless and dismal experience, or will we, in spite of the inevitable suffering, be able to marshal the spiritual forces to face death calmly and triumphantly? How do we prepare ourselves for the great adventure? Having answered these questions perhaps we can be of some help to our patients.

Neither the physicians' nor the clergymen's duties, in this final chapter of a patient's life, can be precisely defined. Each of us is a distinct individual whose body and mind and human experience stamp him as a person set apart, who must be dealt with on the basis of his own merits and demerits. Hence, no universal formula for providing the most effective help is possible. Since there is no rule of thumb to guide us, perhaps the golden rule had better be used. Even this is difficult because, although we have traveled this road with our patients, we have not completed the journey ourselves, and we cannot put ourselves precisely in the position of the patient who is going the whole way. There are, however, a few fundamentals of the physician's role that are basic in every such situation. First, he must make sure that everything that may reasonably be done to effect a cure and make the patient as free of pain as possible has been done. Just as in any clinical situation he has the obligation, as far as the patient's resources will permit, to procure for him the services of any facility or any consultant which he might want for himself were he in the same predicament. Second, he must tell the patient the facts of his physical condition as truthfully and as fully as the patient wishes to know them—always with a liberal admixture of understanding and hope. Just how and how soon this is to be done will vary with each individual, but it is my firm conviction that, with few exceptions, it must be done. Many patients will make it clear that they do not want to be told the whole truth, whether they say it in so many words or not. And, of course, their wishes must be respected. Most will, in the end, have to be told by someone.

The Case for Honesty

Why this insistence on answering the patients' questions honestly? First, human relations are complicated enough without making them more complex by telling lies, which later must be retracted. Second, uncertainty usually is much more difficult to

deal with than the truth, no matter how disturbing the facts
may be. At the same time we must be sure our interpretation of
the facts as we see them is correct. For instance, I once had two
patients with retroperitoneal lymphosarcoma, proved by biopsy,
in the hospital at the same time. The tumors were of approximately the same size and in about the same location, with no
other visible or palpable nodes. The two patients received practically the same course of X-ray therapy. One was dead in three
months. The other lived an active life for nine years.

Thus, what was thought to be a "terminal" illness in both
patients did not prove to be so in one. Ten years ago many of us
felt reasonably certain that patients who had unrelenting azo-
temia of high degree were certain to die within a few months.
Now, with artificial kidneys and renal transplants, we know that
patients formerly doomed to die quickly may have a very much
longer life span. So honesty often must be tempered with optimistic uncertainty.

I was astonished to learn of a survey of the views of a liberal
sampling of physicians on this point, in which more than 70 percent stated that they usually did not inform patients that they
were facing a terminal illness.[1] Some even attempted to justify
giving false information about the diagnosis if they felt patients
were unprepared to accept the truth. For those who hold these
views the reasons may be as cogent as my own for taking the
other point of view. This is an area in which subjective appraisals
are bound to prevail. My own conviction is that never, under
any circumstances, should patients be told untruths. This is the
surest way to destroy the mutual trust and respect which, in the
end, may prove to be the most important therapeutic asset the
physician possesses.

William Bean in his essay "On Death" has stated well the
attitude I share:

> I cannot conceive of the practice of medicine in which there is
> any breach of absolute trust and confidence between patient and
> doctor. A good physician cannot lie to his patient. If the truth be
> bitter, he must help the patient face it. On the other hand, I could
> not bear to practice medicine if I felt obliged always to tell every-

thing I know or think I know. . . . In a materialistic age, in a society which is certainly not notable for individual bravery, independence of thought, or a philosophic attitude, it will not be possible to make a philosopher out of every man during the terminal illness. Perhaps Sir William Jenner's three essential qualities for the medical man will see us through such difficult times: "He must be honest, he must be dogmatic, he must be kind." [2]

Dealing with the Family

Jenner's maxim will do very well in reaching for the proper perspective regarding the patient's family, too. The family member closest to the patient—most often the spouse or parent—must be told the clinical situation, including the prognosis, as fully as the doctor knows it. In this critical time the relationship between patient, family, and physician is, at best, fraught with emotion and it is time-consuming. Since he has been through it before, the doctor must subtly set up some ground rules. First, the warm and friendly attitude of "We are in this thing together" must be created and meant in a very real sense. The patient and the family must be made to know that despite a bleak outlook for care the doctor will see them through, offering understanding and relief of suffering when he cannot offer a cure.

Especially in dealing with patients having metastatic cancer, old ghostly questions almost inevitably come up. "Why was it not discovered in time? If only an operation had been done earlier all this would not have happened. Why should it happen to me, when I have been so careful in my habits and so regular in my examinations?" The feelings of resentment and guilt which prompt such expressed or silent thoughts are terribly tormenting and cannot be ignored. The physician must point out that in any extremely difficult situation one inevitably looks back over his shoulder and asks these same questions. There is usually no justification and certainly no good in patients' attempts to fix the blame on physicians who have previously seen them, on the present medical adviser, or on themselves. Regardless of what has gone before, the situation is there to be faced and the past must be put behind them. From that moment on, the physician should be unyielding in his decision not to listen to hindsight wonderings and recriminations. He must warn the family regarding well-meaning friends whose unsolicited and unreliable advice may provoke panic-striken relatives into spending large amounts of time and money in fruitless visits to other clinics and other physicians. If the patient and his family have had enough confidence in their doctor to put themselves into his hands they should trust him to seek the consultation needed. If they are uncertain about him they should find another physician in whom they are confident, and then follow his advice.

Also, the physician must make it clear that theirs is not the only difficult clinical problem with which he is engaged, and while he intends to help in any constructive way he can and to give information in detail to the relative most directly involved, he is not available for hand-holding and explanations to distant relatives and friends at any hour of the day or night. This may seem to some members of the kindred a heartless attitude, but to the patient himself and to those closest to him it usually is a relief to know that the doctor is in charge and intends to *be* in charge.

The Question of Further Treatment

There are certain questions, such as whether or not special nurses can be afforded, whether possibly risky therapeutic procedures should be done before out-of-town relatives arrive, and the like, which the family obviously must help to decide. But it is not fair or desirable to ask the family or the patient to make decisions regarding clinical management for which their knowledge of the disease or the clinical milieu has not prepared them. This puts a responsibility upon us which as physicians we sometimes long to escape. For example, we are confronted with a patient who, while receiving estrogens for control of cancer of the prostate, is found to have recognizable metastases in the bones of the pelvis. Should bilateral orchiectomy be performed? The physician's decision must consider the profound psychological effect which the procedure may have on the patient as well as the benefit to be anticipated. If his advice is to proceed with the operation, the doctor faces the task of imparting the verdict to the patient in such a way that the physical changes which are sure to ensue will be accepted as worth the good chance for regression of the tumor. He must try as best he can to mitigate the psychological trauma. Should he decide against orchiectomy, he has his own conscience to live with and must have made the decision on the basis of what he thinks his own point of view would be were he in the patient's place. It is quite proper for him to lay the facts before the patient and his family to the extent that they are in position to understand them, but the physician has the obligation to make a decision, whether or not it is accepted.

Other situations may be even more trying. One of them is the discovery of lung or bone metastases in the patient who has had radical mastectomy for cancer of the breast. Should one treat local metastases by radiation as they arise, in the hope of reducing pain and disability, in spite of the knowledge that extensive metastases in other areas are known or strongly suspected of being present—or should he, at once, consider (1) hypophysectomy, with its risk of making the patient a "vegetable" with diabetes insipidus, or (2) adrenalectomy, with its reasonable prospect of prolonging life a few months but carrying the usual risks of causing profound adrenal insufficiency and prolonging suffering? One patient may have no close relatives, be at the end of her financial resources, and be spiritually well-prepared to die. Should the length or the quality of the days remaining to her be the prime consideration? Another patient may have a son to put through college, and have her whole being fixed upon remaining at a remunerative job for that reason, regardless of what happens to her in the way of suffering. Another patient may have the preservation of dignity as her chief goal. She shrinks from androgen therapy or ovariectomy, or either of the ablative procedures previously described, and wants only to be kept as free of pain as is possible, hoping that nothing will be done to prolong her suffering.

All of these attitudes are understandable and must be weighed sympathetically by the physician. Modern medicine's startling

armamentarium for prolonging life makes the problem of inter-
fering with "death from natural causes" extremely difficult. Do
we have the right to interfere significantly with the termination
of physiological processes in a person who seemingly has a hopeless illness and who is a burden to his family and to himself? Or,
as physicians, do we have the obligation always to prolong life
with every means at our disposal? The decision is easy when
dealing with younger persons whose minds are still active and
who still have hope themselves. For older persons in the twilight
of life it is more difficult.

For patients whose only hope for continuation of life is an
organ transplant, is it morally defensible to use as a donor a
relative who is the responsible head of a family of young children, especially if the donor is not an identical twin? These are
all problems for which there is no universally correct answer.
Physicians are beginning thoughtfully to grapple with them, and
they are aware that their colleagues, the clergymen, who are also
interested in the "whole man," must help with the solutions.
Whatever the decision, we must be willing gently to tell the
patient what we think is best, making it clear that some new
therapeutic approach might suddenly be disclosed which could
quickly change the picture. The patient must be made to know
that, regardless of whether he accepts or rejects the decision, the
doctor will continue to help in any way he can as long as the
patient wants his help.

The Provision of Spiritual Support

Having gone this far, is there more that the doctor must do?
Of course, there is. To quote the words of Edward V. Stein,
Ph.D., "He must help the patient grope for values that transcend
both health and survival, to center his being on a faith that
encompasses even his pain and death: In Tillich's words,—'to be
grasped by a power greater than we are.' " [3] This requires some
extraordinary performance on the part of the medical man. And
it is at this point that, unless it has already been accomplished,
he should, if possible, join forces with the clergyman. Quite
often, simply knowing that the physician recognizes the need for

spiritual counsel will be of immense importance to the patient. By his attitude and advice, the physician can make the work of the clergyman easier and more effective. In the same way, the clergyman can support the physician in his efforts.

But the availability of this ally does not absolve us, as doctors, from involvement with our patients' emotional and spiritual problems. In the first place, many patients resist an encounter with the man of God because in their minds his intrusion into the scene so definitely betokens the beginning of the last leg of life's journey. To others, with a deep sense of guilt (And who among us escapes this to some extent?), the clergyman, in some vague way, represents divine judgment which the patient is not yet prepared to face. C. S. Lewis in his penetrating book *The Problem of Pain* says: "It is safe to tell the pure in heart that they shall see God, for only the pure in heart want to."

So, for a time at least, the physician may have to go it alone. Even if the clergyman is warmly welcomed by the patient, the physician cannot abdicate his special role in the patient's spiritual support. Ours is not an ecclesiastical priesthood and we should never attempt to make it so, but it is a priesthood of a sort, nonetheless—one for which medical school has not prepared us. To be prepared for it, somehow each of us must, in his own way, have searched for meaning in his daily tasks. Whether a physician considers himself religious in the conventional sense or not, he must have given some consideration to the universe in which he lives, to the place of man in it, and to the force or mind or God—call it what you will—behind it all. Imperfect as our knowledge and skills may be, we have the matchless opportunity of dealing with human beings in their most profound physical and emotional needs. How we will act in this exquisitely personal relationship will depend upon how we see ourselves in this mighty scheme of things. If, as our religion teaches, there is a touch of the divine in every man—and what perceptive physician who has seen the heroism with which ordinary people meet the greatest calamities can doubt it? The greatest satisfaction we can derive is in helping to unlock the resources that are there to meet the challenge of terminal illness. Our task is not to speak of

heaven or to be the father confessor, unless the patient chooses
to place us in this role. Our task is, rather, to be a friend who is
aware of the road ahead and is willing to go along that road with
the patient, trusting that the human spirit is too precious for
the dissolution of the body to be its final event. Do we or do we
not believe that man has a soul? Do we believe that innocent
babies were brought into the world to grow up and suffer the
awful misfortunes that so many millions of our fellowmen and
their little children suffer, through no error of their own—with
no prospect of anything more significant in their lives or hereafter? Or do we, with the apostle Paul, have the unfaltering hope
of something beyond?

"There is one glory of the sun, and another glory of the
moon, and another glory of the stars; for star differs from star in
glory.

"So is it with the resurrection of the dead. What is sown in
dishonor, it is raised in glory. It is sown in weakness, it is raised
in power. It is sown a physical body, it is raised a spiritual body.
If there is a physical body, there is also a spiritual body.
. . . When the perishable puts on the imperishable, and the mortal puts on immortality, then shall come to pass the saying that is
written:

'Death is swallowed up in victory' (1 Cor. 15:41-44,54)."

I think that even the most skeptical of us will when pressed,
admit to a view akin to that expressed by Mark Twain, "I have
never yet seen what to me seemed an atom of proof that there
is a future life. And yet—I am strongly inclined to expect one." [5]
In discoursing on heaven and death, Sir Thomas Browne, the
seventeenth-century physician, in his *Religio Medici*, says: "I
thank GOD I have not those strait ligaments, or narrow obligations to the World, as to dote on life, or be convulst and tremble
at the name of death. . . . When I take a full view and circle of
my self without this reasonable moderator, and equal piece of
Justice, Death, I do conceive my self the miserablest person
extant. Were there not another life that I hope for, all the
vanities of this World should not intreat a moments breath from

me. . . ." [6] For an interesting view of the prospects and possible content of a life after death, I suggest a perusal of the last chapter of C. S. Lewis' *The Problem of Pain* and *all* of the *Religio Medici.*

Patient Reactions

On rare occasions, persons with terminal illness, on having their suspicions of impending death confirmed, will accept the information with a composure that is hard to comprehend. One woman, who had traveled to many remote parts of the world with her husband and written about them in a fascinating manner, when told—at her request—the findings at her operation for an abdominal malignancy stated: "This *will* be an interesting experience. Don't give me too many sedatives. One dies only once and I don't want to miss any of it. When the time comes for pain killers let me have them—but not now." Her wishes were respected. She went fearlessly to her grave, savoring the full import of the last chapter of her life.

For most patients, however, anxiety beclouds the mind like a fog. Young parents with children to support and put through college see insurmountable financial and social problems ahead. Those whose families have been raised anticipate sympathetically the sorrow of the marriage partner who will be left behind. Almost everyone, upon sensing that his life is drawing to a close, becomes acutely aware of the finality that lies ahead, and the loneliness of the unknown. People who have, for years, lived at a rather superficial level want, for once, desperately to know the deeper significance of life. All want to depart this life with some sense of importance and dignity. And strangely—after the first bewilderment and despair—many seem somehow to attain it.

I quote another passage of the *Religio:* "Thus it is observed, that men sometimes, upon the hour of their departure, do speak and reason above themselves; for then the soul, beginning to be freed from the ligaments of the body, begins to reason like her self, and to discourse in a strain above mortality." [7] Let those who have not been with patients at the bedside in the last days and hours of their final illnesses scoff at the observation of this young physician of three centuries ago. I shall not, for time after time I have seen suddenly appear, in a patient accepting the knowledge of the inevitable, a nobility of spirit that had never been manifest before. It was as if tearing away the veil of uncertainty at the same time released him from fear. He became calm, gentle, considerate of those about him, assuming a new dignity, as if he had already partly crossed the threshold. Not all patients reach this point quickly. It is our duty, and the clergyman's, to help them as they move toward it. Most physicians have not attained the tranquillity of spirit or the felicity of Sir Thomas Browne's words. But we can, at least, stand steadfastly with our patients in this time of trial, letting them know we understand and share their burdens.

Along with the kinds of anxiety mentioned before, many patients have a tormenting sense of guilt upon learning that their final illness is upon them. For some reason, the physical affliction is seen as a punishment for sin. Why this should be, expect for those who actually committed serious crimes, I am not enough of a psychiatrist or theologian to know. I do know it is a devastating experience for the patients who suffer it. With patients who obviously feel the need to unburden their hearts of secrets long repressed, I usually try to retire in favor of the clergyman. He is, in my opinion, much better equipped to deal with the situation. Paul Tournier, who is a physician, says in his book *Guilt and Grace:* "They tell us about their illnesses, their symptoms, their conflicts; in fact, everything they can describe clearly. But they all expect from us something more than our technical attention: not only our sympathy, our personal solicitude or our encouragement but also, in whatever form it may be and perhaps quite unobtrusively, a beam of the divine grace which alone can efface guilt." [8] If the clergyman is not available in such situations, I suppose all we can do is to be good physicians and pray for the "beam of divine grace" which the situation demands. We can point out that all of us are sinners, and usually the worst of us is the least conscious of his guilt. The New Testament is filled with evidence of Christ's compassion for sinners and the assurance that forgiveness and grace and courage to meet life's crises are there for those who want help and pray for it.

In closing, I affirm my hearty agreement with the wise statement of C. S. Lewis: "for the far higher task of teaching fortitude and patience I was never fool enough to suppose myself qualified, nor have I anything to offer my readers except my conviction that when pain is to be borne, a little courage helps more than much knowledge, a little human sympathy more than much courage, and the least tincture of the love of God more than all." [9] If, along with this ingredient and the best medical skills we can acquire, we can attain a love for our fellowmen as well, we have what we need for the ultimate task of ministering to our patients. In the words of Paul, we need this beyond "prophetic powers" and the ability to "understand all mysteries and all knowledge . . ." (1 Cor. 13:2).

HOW CAN A PHYSICIAN PREPARE
HIS PATIENT FOR DEATH?

A thirty-four-year-old woman has Hodgkin's disease. The patient is cognizant of the fact that medication no longer appears to be effective in controlling the progression of this disease. A college graduate and the mother of two children, she has asked a number of questions of her physician and me, which indicate that guidance in this period is desperately desired. How can a physician best prepare his patient for death? What role does a clergyman play in this situation? Would you also discuss these relationships when the patient is a child?

RESPONDENT: *Willard F. Goff, M.D.*

Preparation of a patient for death varies with age, sex, marital status, occupation, country of origin, and religious background.

Children. In Dr. Harvey Cushing's *The Life of Sir William Osler* we find a beautiful picture of the great physician at the bedside of a little girl whose mother wrote:

> He visited our little Janet twice every day from the middle of October until her death a month later, and these visits she looked forward to with a pathetic eagerness and joy. There would be a little tap, low down on the door which would be pushed open and a crouching figure playing goblin would come in, and in a high-pitched voice would ask if the fairy godmother was at home and could he have a bit of tea. Instantly the sick-room was turned into a fairyland, and in fairy language he would talk about the flowers, the birds, and the dolls who sat at the foot of the bed who were always greeted with, 'Well, all ye loves.' In the course of this he

would manage to find out all he wanted to know about the little
patient. . . .

The most exquisite moment came one cold, raw, November
morning when the end was near, and he mysteriously brought out
from his inside pocket a beautiful red rose carefully wrapped in
paper, and told how he had watched this last rose of summer
growing in his garden and how the rose had called out to him
as he passed by, that she wished to go along with him to see his
little lassie. That evening we all had a fairy teaparty, at a tiny
table by the bed, Sir William talking to the rose, his 'little lassie,'
and her mother in a most exquisite way; and presently he slipped
out of the room just as mysteriously as he had entered it, all
crouched down on his heels; and the little girl understood that
neither fairies nor people could always have the colour of a red
rose in their cheeks, or stay as long as they wanted to in one place,
but that they nevertheless would be very happy in another home
and must not let the people they left behind, particularly their
parents, feel badly about it; and the little girl understood and was
not unhappy.[1]

I would never deliberately tell a child he was going to die.
Neither would I lie if the question was asked.

For young children, it is enough to explain that God is our
loving heavenly Father, who, like our earthly father, will always
take care of us, no matter where we live or where we go. Most
everyone likes to take a trip or journey to a far country. God
has promised to go with us and stay with us wherever we go.
Sometimes our bodies get tired and can no longer work. Our
heart stops beating and we go to sleep. But the real person is still
living.

Perhaps there is nothing more important to a dying child
than to have a parent or physician hold his hand. The child
learns to identify his parent or physician with his image of God.

Adults. "Physicians have two duties: (1) to preserve life, and
(2) to prevent or ameliorate suffering." [2] However, as death approaches, the patient looks to his physician for help. Preparing
an adult for death depends largely on his background and recep-
tivity. Regardless of the patient's belief in a hereafter, the physician must inspire hope. This hope may include hope that the
medicine will still effect a cure, and hope that another type of

treatment may be tried. "The physician who refuses to adopt an attitude of hopelessness and despair toward patients with advanced cancer may succeed in adding worthwhile years to the lives of some of those otherwise doomed to early and miserable death, and on rare occasions may bring about cure." [3]

"Our task is not to speak of heaven or to be the father confessor, unless the patient chooses to place us in the role. Our task is, rather to be a friend who is aware of the road ahead and is willing to go along that road with the patient, trusting that the human spirit is too precious for the dissolution of the body to be its final event." [4] The physician "is far more than a mechanic whose business it is to prolong life." [5]

There is a hospital in Dublin called the "Hospital for the Incurables." To my mind, no physician has sufficient knowledge to tell his patient that his condition is incurable or hopeless or that there is no life after death. We must never tell a patient how much longer he has to live. It is just possible that he might outlive us.

The sincere physician must inspire positive thoughts in the patient, i.e., faith in the doctor, nurse, and others entrusted to his care; faith in a future life which will be free of pain and suffering; and faith that life is the preparation of the soul for eternity.

The Orthodox Jew believes in a bodily resurrection as is found in the Old Testament (cf. Isa. 26:19; Dan. 12:2; Ezek. 37:5; and Ps. 23:4).

The Liberal Jew does not believe in physical resurrection, but he does believe in the continuity of life. Rabbi Raphael H. Levine, Temple de Hirsch, Seattle, believes "that in God's world there is no death. There is only life on different levels of experience." [6]

For the Christian, a future life with God is a certainty because of Christ's resurrection and his promise: "I am the resurrection and the life; he who believes in me, though he die, yet shall he live, and whoever lives and believes in me shall never die" (John 11:25-26).

THE PATIENT WITH
A FATAL ILLNESS
—TO TELL OR NOT TO TELL

A sixty-two-year-old man has carcinoma of the lung with wide-spread metastases. His wife and his twenty-year-old son, who is now in college, know the diagnosis, but the patient has not been told. What are your guidelines for "telling" or "not telling"? Would it be helpful if the clergyman of the family were told of the entire scientific background by the physician or should this information reach the clergyman via the family?

RESPONDENT: *Arthur H. Becker, Ph.D.*

If we accept the proposition that the matrix of relationships within which a person lives is vital and to a large degree constitutive of his existence as a person, then we need to be aware of the effect that critical information in the minister's or physician's possession may have on these vital relationships. The rule "be absolutely honest with the patient" does not meet all the requirements of a Christian ethic—nor does it meet the professional requirements of the physician "to do no harm." Rather, the physician, as well as any other professional person who is involved with critical information in a person's life, strives to be honest in such a way that the truth is most constructive or least destructive to the person in his relationships.

Communicating the information which the physician holds in stewardship requires that he deal with such issues as these:

1. How genuinely and with what integrity are the patient and his family able to respond and relate to each other in *the present state of affairs?*

2. What effect does withholding the information from the patient have on his relationships with his family? on the family's relationship with the patient? on the patient's relationship with the physician and the converse? How does it affect the patient's own self-understanding?

3. Will *withholding or sharing* the information set up barriers and facades between the patient, his family, his physician, etc., behind which lurk fear, guilt, and anxiety, thus destroying or weakening the relations between the patient, his family, and the patient and his physician?

4. Are the relationships between the family and the patient sufficiently strong and open so that sharing the reality of an impending death will not shatter or destroy them? How can the patient and his family constructively utilize the information that might be shared?

In many instances the decision to "tell" should be delayed until the family can be strengthened so that they will be able to "talk" with the patient about his feelings with integrity. This may be the task of the physician, or it may be the task of the clergyman. In some instances, the channels of communication are so blocked with conflicts that they must first be resolved where possible, before any further burden is placed upon them.

5. Are the members of the patient's family and the patient himself fully able to assimilate and in a healthy manner rationalize the information? With children a very important consideration is the ability simply to understand the information, and to be able to understand the meaning of death itself. Where such ability is lacking, communicating the information serves no useful purpose. With adults, this involves not only rational abilities, but the willingness to face the information and to deal creatively with the implications of it. As a general rule, physicians have waited for the patient himself to ask a more or less direct question before sharing terminal diagnostic information. This question is presumed evidence of the willingness of the patient to deal with it and the capabilities to do so.

As a hospital chaplain, I have found, however, that the patient hesitates to ask the physician for a variety of reasons: a fear of displaying lack of trust in the doctor, the feeling that the doctor himself is threatened by the possibility of death, or the feeling that the doctor either does not have time or is not willing to sit down and "work through" the implications of the information with the patient. Accordingly, the question "Am I going to die?" is addressed to the chaplain. Properly, he should not answer this since it is a medical matter; he should in turn confer with the physician. In many instances then, the two in concert determine the best course in answering the question.

6. Will a change in the situation from the patient's present state of awareness as to his prognosis bring about improvements in the matrix of relationships in which the patient lives?

It is fairly commonly held that the terminal patients who are conscious and at all perceptive seem to "know" that they are going to die, even though they have not been told. If we assume that this is the case, is the patient struggling in relative isolation with a burden (either real or imagined) which could be eased if he had more accurate information and felt free to share it with someone else? Through such sharing, could he be helped to deal with his situation with less anxiety? On the other hand, the patient frequently "knows" but there is no evidence that this knowledge, though not shared with anyone, in any way disturbs the relationships he has with physician, family, or friends. In such instances, nothing constructive seems to be gained by imparting the critical information.

7. One of the issues the clergyman is always concerned with is the patient's relationship to God. It is sometimes put in this form: does the patient need to make his peace with God? The assumption is that he will not do so without the added impetus of knowing that his life is soon to end. This is not entirely healthy, obviously. Ideally, the patient's relationships with God are so open and viable that he is concerned to be at peace with God whether he will live one day or a hundred years. This is often not the case, however. The patient's personal relationship with God must be considered vital along with the whole constellation of human relationships in which he lives. Normally, where the patient has a viable and open relationship with his

church and clergyman, the clergyman should be informed of the diagnosis so that he may be able to provide what assistance is necessary in bringing about a redeemed relationship with God. It is frequently the family itself that shares such information with the minister, although the physician may do so under the provisions for "professional or privileged communication." The clergyman can also be helpful to the physician in arriving at a decision whether to inform the patient on the basis of the previously mentioned categories. The clergyman also can be very helpful in supporting the patient in his situation and working through the implications of what he is facing.

There are, of course, other prudential issues involved, such as making a will and disposal of property, which must be considered as well.

RESPONDENT: *Avery D. Weisman, M.D.*

Whether or not to tell a patient with a fatal illness about his prognosis is almost always the first question asked by families and physicians; yet, it may be the least important part of the total treatment program. Few families spontaneously prefer that their ailing kin be told directly, but this initial response should not be accepted as final. Families often need more help in accepting the likelihood of death in the foreseeable future than does the patient himself. If we were truly to operate in accord with what is already understood about the psychology of dying patients, we would tell the patient first, using the qualifications described below, and then ask the patient what and how the family should be told.

For the sake of simplicity, I shall avoid rhetoric and rationalization, and only state the principles on which these conclusions are based.

The central question is not whether or not to tell a patient about his dim outlook, but *who* shall tell, *how much* to tell, *what* to tell, *how* to tell, *when* to tell, and *how often* to tell.

Who shall tell? Telling a patient is only the beginning, certainly not the end. It is not a painful task to be gotten out of the way, or to be relinquished gladly to someone else, such as to a minister or another family member. For everyone concerned, it is a genuine opportunity to reaffirm the reality of a human relationship. For the physician, it is an obligation and probably a necessary step, if the patient is to have a reasonably tranquil terminal period. Physicians who are most reluctant to talk about death with their patients are sometimes those who are also most reluctant to order sufficient analgesics and tranquilizers in the terminal stage. This suggests that, on both counts, these doctors avoid direct confrontation with death, perhaps to spare anguish for themselves, not for their patients.

How much to tell? Telling a patient about his terminal illness is certainly not like giving him neutral information. A patient should be told only as much as he can use and absorb at the moment. A doctor should give information gradually, often over a series of visits, watching for individual responses and inquiries, allowing for idiosyncratic reactions, and being prepared to modulate the conversation to correct for unexpected complications. Rules and standard policies only approximate the facts; individual variations are the only rules.

What to tell? Most patients already have a fairly accurate intimation about the trend of illness by the time the physician and family get around to telling them. When a patient denies concern, he usually does so in order to preserve a relationship with someone on whom he is dependent, and cannot afford to alienate—and this includes the physician taking care of him. It is by no means rare for terminal patients to conceal the extent of their awareness, lest the doctor or family become upset!

Initially, most patients should be advised of the doctor's findings *and the treatment planned.* Frankness does not mean hopelessness, nor does unrealistic denial do more than foster temporary reassurance. At the beginning, the patient need not be told more than the facts of his illness. His doctor's directness should convey a more important, nonverbal message that he will not be abandoned. Gratuitous reassurances, overly precise predictions, and philosophical precepts are to be avoided.

How to tell? Plenty of time is needed for a significant human interchange. Information that involves a strong emotion can be given openly, but in the direction of the patient's strengths. Avoid technical terms, because the doctor's concern about the histological type of tumor, for example, may not be the patient's concern. The predominant concerns of dying patients are usually not with the fact of dying, but with fears of isolation, abandonment, intractable pain, or of being sent off to a nursing home to languish and die. The physician, then, should be prepared for responses that seem to be accepting but are not, for delayed responses, and for anxieties not literally expressed that actually refer to something else. As a rule, the doctor cannot recognize the difference between true acceptance and outright denial without knowing the patient for a long time. Simple sincerity is a better guide to *how to tell* than are clichés or standard formulas which tend to protect the doctor without helping the patient.

When to tell? Although families may at first protest about giving the patient any information, lest he give up, become insane, or commit suicide, let them know that these reactions are decidedly uncommon. If the patient does not already know or suspect, families must be assured that soon it will be impossible and even undesirable to keep the "secret." Let them know also that dissimulation risks alienation and abandonment long before the patient is, in fact, ready to die. Families who have been the least accessible to the patient during health are often those who show the most opposition to telling the patient the truth about his illness.

How often to tell? After the initial step of candor and confidence has been taken, subsequent discussions become easier. Because communication is uncluttered with rationalizations and unnecessary apologies, patients can be told about new symptoms and why older symptoms have not responded to treatment. Openness means that patients are told that they will have enough medication to reduce pain and that they will be consulted when procedures which merely prolong survival are being considered. By damaging a patient's sense of being a person, unnecessary procedures may inflict more suffering and exact a greater price than the biological extension of life in terms of days or weeks can justify.

Few patients persist in talking about dying. They accommodate to awareness of death, especially in the advanced stages of illness, and still more when they can face death with their doctor's help. Availability of the doctor leads to acceptance by the patient, even though acceptance may come gradually. Conversely, efforts by the doctor to encourage denial in the patient may lead to the doctor's denial of the patient as a person. After all, the physician's prime consideration, once death can no longer be postponed, should be to help the patient live as effectively as possible until he dies.

SHOULD THE CANCER PATIENT BE TOLD?

Most clinicians have experienced the dilemma of whether to tell a patient with incurable malignancy the true diagnosis. A comparison among physicians is not uncommon in the hospital cafeteria or during medical meetings. However, I would be very interested in knowing the opinion of the clergy regarding their views of the advisability of disclosing or withholding the prognosis from the patient. I am thinking particularly of a fifty-three-year-old woman with carcinoma of the breast (and metastases) who is frightened by the word "cancer" because of the implication of pain and suffering associated with this term. Nevertheless, I suspect that the patient does have the fortitude and the desire for a more candid discussion of the gravity of her illness.

RESPONDENT: *Rt. Rev. Msgr. James G. Wilders*

Some years ago the Office of Cancer Teaching and Research of Marquette University School of Medicine sponsored a symposium including the legal, psychiatric, and moral aspects of this question.

On the legal side, the point particularly stressed was that a physician could be held legally liable if his failure to inform the patient of the nature of his disease would be a cause of danger to the patient. An interesting case was cited of a man who had made a large investment and who later sued his physician on the grounds that if the physician had revealed to him his true condition, he would not have embarked on this perilous business venture. Another obvious case of legal liability concerned costly deception of a patient by holding out false hopes of recovery and thus inducing the patient to undergo expensive treatments which the physician should have recognized to be useless.

Psychiatrists stressed the need of estimating the probable reaction of the patient before telling him he has cancer, and they insisted that the physician must avoid an approach and the use of terms that might create anxiety. It was pointed out that the very word "cancer" fills many people with dread and that the discovery that they have cancer might be the occasion of a severe depression. The psychiatrists would be in favor of a general educational policy which would help people to view the prospect of having cancer with more calm, but they believe that at present, when the danger of creating harmful anxiety is so great, the problem of notifying the patient defies general rules and must be looked upon as a decidedly individualistic one.

In this regard, the duty of telling the patient of his critical condition so that he can prepare well for death does not necessarily include the obligation of telling him the precise nature of his illness. For instance, there is the case of the devout Catholic mother who died of cancer, apparently without ever having suspected the character of the disease. But she expected to die, and she was always prepared to go, as she put it, "when the Lord wanted to take me." Since she did not ask what was wrong with her, her physician and her family agreed to say nothing about the precise nature of the ailment because they thought this information might induce an unfavorable psychological reaction by creating an uneasy anticipation of pain. They came to this decision only after they had made sure that she was entertaining no false hope of recovery.

At the Marquette symposium, the moralists' view of the problem can be summarized along the legal and psychiatric lines already indicated. In the first place, the moralist would certainly agree with the lawyer that to damage a patient through deceit is wrong. It is not merely a judicial fault but also a moral fault to take money under false pretenses or to conceal the true state of affairs from a patient, with the knowledge that he will be led by false hopes to damage himself financially. But the moralist would not limit the consideration of "damage to the patient" to the mere material or monetary sphere. He would think equally, even primarily, in terms of spiritual damage.

It is important for every religious-minded Christian and Jew to prepare for death. For the Catholic, the effect of the last sacraments must not be minimized. These should be administered when he is conscious, if possible, remembering that one of the effects of these sacraments is peace of soul and another, return to physical health if God so wills.

I know from my fifteen years of experience going day after day from bedside to bedside in the New York Hospital that many devout people expressed regret at the time of last sacraments that they had not been notified earlier so they could have spent time more profitably and accumulated richer merits from heaven.

All these things must be considered, and I think that they can best be considered where the hospital has a full chaplaincy program for patients of all faiths, where doctors and chaplains learn to work closely with one another and to have confidence in one another, truly, where the clergy-doctor team works in perfect cooperation and coordination.

THE DYING PATIENT AND
HIS FAMILY

Peter F. Regan, M.D.

The keystone to the management of the episode of death is the recognition that death is a crisis—for the patient, for his family, and for the physician. If the physician accepts his responsibility in directing this crisis toward a peaceful outcome for the patient and a healthy outcome for the family, he can follow certain procedures. In following these and in planning appropriate strategy, he can usually achieve satisfactory ends and prevent a tragic death from becoming a disaster.

It is characteristic of medicine that effective, coordinated action depends on an understanding of the basic process being treated. Whether the physician deals with a ruptured appendix, an infarcted myocardium, or a fractured radius, the pattern is the same—effective treatment follows understanding. Without such understanding, argument and confusion reign, while the patient suffers.

Nowhere is the need for understanding of the basic process more evident than in the management of the episode of death.

To be sure, it is beyond our human capacities to have a full understanding of each death. On the other hand, our knowledge of this process is sufficiently detailed so that steps can be taken to improve our approaches to a significant degree. It will be the purpose of this communication to explore something of this knowledge, and to indicate how it can be applied, as the physician deals with the patient and his family, before, during, and after the episode of death.

Death as a Crisis

As soon as death is considered as one of a number of natural processes, it is apparent that death has in it the prime element of these processes—the element of crisis. In every sense, the time of death is a crisis for the patient, for his family, and for the physician.

For the patient. The elements of crisis that death holds, for the patient, are well recognized.[1] He is assaulted by pain and disease, by the loss of dignity as a human being, and by increasing estrangement from his family and friends. Will he succumb to the fear and pain, will he erect pathological defenses like denial, revenge, or suicide; or will he forge a peaceful, calm death? That is his crisis.

For the family. The family's crisis is more varied. The family must stand by the patient at the end of life, giving him support despite their own suffering. After death, the family must come to grips with the shock of loss and the need to express grief. Finally, through successful mourning, the members must regroup, and face the world, renewed.

For the physician. The physician's crisis, in death, is perhaps the most complex. It is his responsibility to direct the interplay of forces toward a constructive outcome. Just as he presides at the coming in, so also does he preside at the going out. In presiding, he must manage to help the patient achieve the most peaceful death possible, and help the family go through each of its crises successfully.

The Physician's Attitude

As many great physicians have pointed out, the key to success in managing the crisis of death lies in the physician's attitude.[2] Can he be satisfied with the "successful management" of a death?

The chief means toward achieving the attitude lies in the physician's recognition of his total responsibility; he is far more than a mechanic whose business it is to prolong life. His classic role in society is that of a responsible person to whom the patient can turn, with trust and confidence, for advice, as well as for technical help. This role does not call for heroic measures and frantic maneuvers once hope is lost, nor does it allow the physician to feel defeated when death supervenes. Once the optimal physical measures have been carried out, the physician's role is to help patient and family deal with the outcome, good or bad, despite the difficulty of maintaining his efforts in an increasingly discouraging situation.[3] With such efforts, the crises have every opportunity to be resolved satisfactorily.

With such a therapeutic attitude about death, the physician may follow certain clear patterns in managing this situation.

Techniques in Management

The use of skilled honesty. In most instances, the physician and the patient have advance warning that death is approaching. Such a warning will have many degrees of certainty of time. Whatever the situation, however, the physician must resolve the enigmatic problem: how to inform the patient of the grim situation without injuring him.

The issue of informing the patient about a grave prognosis has received much attention. Clearly, the matter is one which involves the personal attitudes of physicians and for which there is no absolute answer.[4] Certainly, if the patient is not informed, his relatives must be made aware of the situation.

If the patient is to be informed of approaching death, the physician must go about the task in a fashion which will help, not injure, the patient. In doing so, the physician should bear in mind the following points:

1. The information should be provided in an open-ended fashion. Thus, while the physician may indicate what his professional opinion is, he can, at the same time, indicate that this opinion is no more and no less than an educated estimate of probabilities, and is not to be taken as infallible.

2. The information should be phrased positively.[5] Thus, the patient can be informed of his reasonable minimal life expectancy rather than of the probable date of his death.

3. Once the information has been expressed in an open-ended and positive fashion, further explication can depend on the patient. The patient may or may not wish more information;

the family almost invariably will. Here, the physician can put his information at their disposal as seems indicated.

4. Once the information has been provided, the physician must not insist on repeating it. Many patients, after having absorbed the initial open-ended and positive expression, will prefer never to mention the matter again, to go on with a tacit understanding with the physician. Others will want repeated discussions. The wise physician will follow the indications provided by the patients in this regard.

Mobilizing support before death. As the time of death approaches, the patient is beset by feelings of loneliness and estrangement, as well as by apprehension about the future, and by the ravages of his illness. Naturally, the physician will deal with the latter in direct and effective fashion.[6] For loneliness and apprehension, he can truly set a model for the family to follow. There are several techniques which he may utilize:

First, in dealing with the patient, he can avoid the dangers of oversolicitousness, or false reassurance. Everything *isn't* "all right"; neither is everything lost. The physician can help the patient in establishing a fair appraisal of what is possible and what is not possible in the situation, so that he can obtain the full satisfactions which are available in the period of life remaining to him.

Second, instructions to the family should include urging that they neither give way to excessive emotional displays in the presence of the patient, nor, on the other hand, conceal their legitimate concern. Like the physician, whom they can imitate, the family should be realistic and concerned in their approach, thereby enabling themselves to render the strongest support to the patient.

Further, the physician can encourage the family to call other resources which can help to relieve the patient's anxiety and apprehension. Most notably, the patient's minister can provide immeasurable comfort in the lonely hours that precede death.

The physician's assumption of authority. In this age of technical advances, no one is more thoroughly familiar with the elaborate techniques available for prolonging life than is the physician. By the same token, no one is more aware of the futility of these measures, in many instances, than the physician. Certainly, we have all seen instances of an *organism* maintained alive after all hope for the *person* returning to life was irretrievably gone.

There is no sight so tragic as that of the family asked by the physician whether he should continue heroic measures; the family, in such a situation, has no way of knowing what is right, and the physician is abnegating the basic responsibilities which are his.

It is the physician's duty instead, to use his wisdom and clinical judgment in recommending that the family utilize all the techniques of modern medicine, as far as these are likely to be helpful and effective, but to abstain from these recommendations when the threshold of effectiveness is past.

Providing an opportunity for ventilation. When death has occurred, the family is in a state of emotional shock—whether from sudden and unexpected loss, from relief of prolonged agony, or from grief. At this time, too, the physician is usually tired and saddened. It is exactly at this point, however, that it becomes his burden not to turn away and seek his own peace, but to turn toward the family. He needs to explain to them what has happened in simple and sympathetic words, and to give them the opportunity of easing their own suffering. Almost every family needs to be reassured, at this time, that everything was done (i.e., that *they* did everything they could), that the patient's suffering was minimal, and that it is now over. Depending on the family, they need to weep with the physician, to complain, or to obtain reassurance and support. A minimum of ten minutes spent in this constructive effort can provide a suitable conclusion to the management of the crisis of death and can turn the family toward their job of reestablishing their new integrity and working toward the future.

THEORIES OF ETHICS AND MEDICAL PRACTICE

Chauncey D. Leake, Ph.D., Sc.D.

There is much popular and professional confusion over ethics. It is important at once to realize that "ethics" is not a single agreed-upon system of moral conduct, but rather that there are many ethics and many theories of how it is best to behave. In medical practice the confusion is heightened by the frequent tendency to think of etiquette as ethics.

Social and Professional Control of Medicine

Current technical advance in biomedical endeavor, such as organ transplantation and fertility control, has brought a bewildering shift in our understanding of moral problems associated with medical practice. No longer are there solid and immutable absolutes for our comfort. We are increasingly facing the necessity of making wise judgments promptly on the spot, on the basis of as many of the factors in the immediate situation as we can recognize and with as full an understanding as possible of the consequences of our conduct.

From antiquity there has been confusion between medical etiquette on the one hand and medical ethics on the other. Medical etiquette has generally been concerned with the personal appearance, dignified comportment, and courteous interprofessional relations of practicing members of the health professions. Ancient Chinese, Hindu, Graeco-Roman, Medieval, and eighteenth-century writings of medical leaders repeatedly emphasized the social importance of maintaining gentlemanly dignity in medical practice. Even the famed code of "Medical Ethics," finally issued in 1803 by Thomas Percival (1740–1804) for the guidance of the Manchester members of the health professions, is more of an Emily Post-style guide to proper social conduct than it is a discussion of basic moral problems to help in the daily judgments necessary in medical practice which so often determine the sort of life or death that may follow in individual patients. When the American Medical Association was organized in 1847 for the purpose of improving the character of medical education and medical practice in our country, Percival's code was adopted without the physicians realizing that it is concerned with etiquette and not ethics. The use of the phrase "code of medical ethics" has been responsible for much professional as well as popular confusion between the real moral problems of medicine, with which theories of ethics are concerned, and mere etiquette, with which theories of ethics are only incidentally significant.

The moral aspects of medical practice have come under social and professional control. The earliest legal code of which we have record was that instituted by Hammurabi around 2000 B.C. for the guidance of the people of his Sumerian Empire. This code set fees to be charged for medical service and invoked the lex talionis principle (an eye for an eye, a tooth for a tooth). It was a tough code. Yet the physician might ransom his life or a part of his body if he had killed or injured a corresponding part of his patient. This was the origin of the malpractice suit with the payments it might entail. Social control of medical practice was intended in A.D. 1222 when the Emperor Frederick II of the Holy Roman Empire issued an edict that only those persons could treat the sick for a fee who had passed an examination for proficiency set by the faculty of the school of Salerno. This was the pioneering state-licensing regulation for medicine, and it has been followed by state systems ever since. Further social regulation of the practice of medicine seems to be underway, often with unpleasant economic aspects.

Professional control of the practice of medicine has been followed from the time of Hippocrates (fifth century B.C.) to the present, by means of professional organizations and by continued exhortation to follow high moral standards. The Hippocratic physicians left for us the inspiration of the *Oath, Law, Decorum,* and *Precepts.* These have been responsible in large part for promoting and maintaining high moral principles of medical practice. There has often been a lurking suspicion that they are not quite satisfactory for application to current affairs. The Geneva Modification of the Hippocratic Oath has been an attempt to update the document and make it relevant to our times, at least in respect to human experimentation or genocide. The Hippocratic Oath still interdicts abortion, but now problems involving abortion are becoming of serious moral significance. On the other hand, the injunction to secrecy regarding the personal affairs of patients is still generally followed. Even here, however, there now seem to be situations in which such secrecy is not justified, either from the standpoint of the privacy of individual patients, or of social or public welfare.

The Moral Problems of Medicine

Joseph Fletcher, the distinguished theologian, currently raises some of the basic moral questions arising in medical practice. These concern abortion, fertility control, gene manipulation, euthanasia, the right of a patient to know the truth, and miscegenation. These difficulties have been with us from antiquity.

Public attitudes toward abortion are changing in the face of clear evidence that certain diseases in pregnancy may cause serious malformations in unborn children. Abortion might be thought of as merely a more humane way of disposing of malformed infants than the ancient method of exposure of children not wanted. Fertility control, in the face of the fulfillment of the Malthusian prophecy, is essential for our species, whether popes approve or not. The problem of euthanasia is related to the problem of the right of a patient to know the truth or the right of a patient to die when there is no chance for recovery. Our current biomedical knowledge permits us to keep patients alive indefinitely, even when they may have no functioning brain at all. There, as in problems associated with organ transplantation, we need agreement on a satisfactory definition of death which must be in accord with our modern scientific information. The attempt by the Harvard Medical group to furnish such a definition met with surprising public acceptance. The hard facts of biological organization among humans is slowly settling the problem of miscegenation, whether we like it or not. More important for moral judgment among physicians in the future will be genetic control.

There are six specific biomedical advances that raise grave moral questions. These are (1) organ transplantation, including the use of organ and tissue banks or artificial organs, in which conflicting ethical principles motivate the recipients, the donors, the respective families, the members of the health professions, and the public; (2) hemodialysis, in which economic factors bring up the old conflict between community and individual desires and responsibilities; (3) genetic control through gene manipulation, which is still experimental at the level of molecular organization of living material, but which has frightening future potential as forecast so vividly by Aldous Huxley in *Brave New World;* (4) artificial insemination, where there is legal difficulty over considerations of illegitimacy, inheritance rights, and family relationships; (5) the alteration of environments by destruction of natural conditions or by pollution of airs and waters, which involves our responsibilities to maintain a healthy world for our descendants; and (6) the development of new chemicals, designed for specific use as antibiotics, contraceptives, growth regulators, or as agents for cancer control or for altering mood and behavior, where the moral issues involve human experimentation as well as the purposes of ultimate use.

The moral aspects of problems associated with current biomedical advance involve ethical theory. They are not concerned with mere etiquette. We can take for granted the guidelines developed by Percival and the AMA to assure courteous conduct and decent interpersonal relations between members of the health professions and services and between them and their pa-

tients. We cannot as easily dismiss the conflicting points of view
raised by the various ethical theories.

Ethical Theories

It should at once be realized that there are many ethics. They
are the various answers which have been proposed since olden
days to a basic question, "What is good?" These various answers
are tentative and relative, quite like the various answers to those
other basic questions raised by the Greeks, "What is true?" and
"What is beautiful?"

The general moral problem involves a fundamental question,
"What are we living for?" This includes consideration of our
motives, our actions, our conduct, our interpersonal relations,
our moods, and our behavior.

It was early recognized that in order to accomplish effectively whatever purpose one might have in mind, it would be
wise to have as much sound knowledge about the various factors
in that purpose as possible. This brought up the basic problem
of "What is true?" Again there are many answers. These com-
prise the various logics. Examples are the long dominant Aris-
totelian logic of deduction from revealed or assumed axioms (as
in Euclidean geometry); an inductive logic as devised by Francis
Bacon in the seventeenth century; and the symbolic logic designed by Whitehead and Russell. The great success of scientific
logic has been due to its method for independent verification.
This gives the most satisfactory foundation for success in the
accomplishment of individual or social purposes.

In order to apply effectively the verifiable knowledge we may
have of ourselves and of our environment to the accomplishment
of specific or general purposes, it is necessary to use judgment in
selecting that information which is fitting or appropriate to the
particular purpose in mind, and then to try to apply that knowledge with its consequences to achieving the goal. This is a matter
of aesthetics. Thus, physicians have the general purpose of trying
to restore or to maintain optimum health in individual patients.
It requires much judgment to select from the great store of verifiable information on health and disease that which is appro-

priate and possibly helpful to the particular patient involved. Judgment is acquired chiefly by careful study of the humanities and the arts. Since judgment is so essential a part of medical practice, it is customary to refer to medicine as a science and as an art.

The various ethics try to win public approval about individual and social goals and purposes, about motives, about guides for conduct as well as about factors which influence interpersonal relations or which may determine moods and behavior. The disciplines of psychology and sociology are thus often more involved in ethical discussions than are other biological sciences. Recent developments in neurophysiology, however, may make this field dominant even in psychology and sociology.

Part of our difficulty concerning ethical problems results from the conditions of organizational levels of living material. Through lack of adequate understanding we tend to confuse factors which may operate at an *individual* level of biological organization with those operating at a *social* level. Individual "good" may not always coincide with social "good," even if some of our hippies and yippies would want it so. Much ethical theory is concerned with attempts to harmonize these often divergent conditions of individual and social welfare.

In a rather formal, conventionalized, and often ritualistic manner, the earliest moral exhortations were usually imposed by community action, often with the force of religious fervor, and were mostly based on the experiences of tribal living. The Mosaic Decalogue with its categorical "shalls" and "shall nots" is a typical example. By the fifth century b.c. there was sufficient sophistication among the Greeks for them to propose that our prime purpose in living is to get as much personal pleasure as possible and that our behavior should be directed toward obtaining maximum personal happiness. This is the ultimate in individual good. It is the ethic of *hedonism*. Actually it is not quite as simple as it may sound. Practical circumstances intervene. Adjustments to others become necessary for any happiness to be obtained at all, for anyone. Thus, a conscious enlightened *individualism* may emerge, as Warner Fite suggests.[1]

While hedonism takes into account the desires and purposes of individuals, the broader social good was emphasized by Plato. He pointed out that individual happiness is dependent upon social welfare. In Platonic *social idealism,* the prime good is the welfare of the social group, to which an individual belonging is expected to sacrifice his or her own personal welfare, voluntarily. This became the conventional Judeo-Christian ethic, and it is also, to our confusion, the ethical principle behind communism, an ideology which Christian Americans are not supposed to tolerate.

Various attempts have been made to find an effective compromise between hedonism and Platonic social idealism. Aristotle, the pupil of Plato, proposed that we would be wise to act in such a way as to harmonize most fittingly with our environments. Almost in anticipation of Darwinian principles, this harmony ethic suggests survival values on the basis of adaptation.

While Immanuel Kant in the eighteenth century made a huge intellectual effort to derive a "categorical imperative" as a guiding ethical principle, it is difficult to understand and impossible to follow, since the decisions which it would entail are usually beyond our capacity or ability.

Another attempt to get a working compromise between hedonism and Platonic social idealism was made by Jeremy Bentham, and extended by Herbert Spencer and John Stuart Mill in the nineteenth century, under the term "utilitarianism." This is the principle of striving to obtain the "greatest good for the greatest number." As Warner Fite has indicated, this turns out to be a calculated hedonism.[2]

William James, the great Boston physician-psychologist, advocated the ethical principle of pragmatism. This suggests, again along evolutionary lines, that whatever works out satisfactorily on the basis of trial or experimentation is good. This is the position frequently, if unconsciously, taken by members of the health professions and services in adaptation to the particular situation confronting them in their respective practices. Pragmatism is the professional ethic, generally.

More recently such biologists as Julian Huxley, S. J. Holmes, and C. H. Waddington have become interested in a possible scientific basis for an ethic. This seems to be most readily derivable from evolutionary and survival considerations. This trend, starting with Edwin Grant Conklin about four decades ago, has been greatly accelerated by the tough moral problems raised by the applications of nuclear energy.

Actually, some thirty years ago, at a pleasant Sunday afternoon seminar in the Santa Cruz redwoods in California, a group of scientists made an attempt to induce a naturally operating ethic which would function on a basis of survival factors and which would be operative, whether or not we recognized it or whether or not we like it. This was worked out by Edwin Grant Conklin, the distinguished biologist, who had taught me at Princeton, and who then was President of the American Association for the Advancement of Science; Judson Herrick, the wise and brilliant neurologist of the University of Chicago; Olaf Larsell, the great neuroanatomist of the University of Oregon; and myself. It was later critically examined by my friend Patrick Ronnell, an outstanding philosopher, now at Texas Western University.

After considering the wealth of common experience in the everyday interplay of differing personalities, we used inductive logical methods to develop from many particulars a generality which seems to be naturally operative in governing interpersonal relations, and perhaps also in guiding the motives, purposes, and moods associated with them. This general principle may be stated thus: *the probability of the survival of a relationship between individuals, or between groups of individuals, increases with the extent to which that relationship is mutually satisfying.*

If we assume the validity of this principle, an important consequence follows: if either party to a relationship wishes the relationship to continue, it is necessary to do whatever is possible to make the relationship satisfying to the other party. This is reminiscent of what is called the Golden Rule. A significant concept in this naturally operating principle is that of satisfaction. At the time we proposed this ethical principle, we did not have as much verifiable information as we now possess about the biological background for the emotional sense of satisfaction.

Biologically, as Paul MacLean indicates and as many studies by others confirm, our purpose in living seems to be dependent upon two built-in drives which originate in two groups of cells in our primitive brain-stem limbic systems. These drives direct us toward satisfaction in a continual cyclical recurrent search for food (needed for self-preservation), and in the postpuberty search for sex (needed for species preservation).[3] The biological answer to that ancient question of "What do we live for?" seems to be to obtain recurring satisfaction from the cyclical recurring drives for food and for sex.

These basic drives for food and for sex become subject to extensive individual conditioning in different ways in different people, in accordance with differing experiences, and the conditioning may proceed not only reflexly, but at different levels of consciousness. Further, these basic biological drives may be variously sublimated in different people so that satisfactions may be obtained from directing these drives toward fame, fortune, fantasy, or fun.

Failure to get satisfaction from these built-in drives for food or sex, or their conditional surrogates, may result in psychodynamisms of serious consequence. If a person is conscious that the satisfaction he is seeking may possibly not come, he is in an uneasy state of anxiety. A little anxiety is probably good for us in our competitive world. But if the feeling goes to the point of realizing the probability of losing the desired satisfaction, frustration comes on. This has a peculiar tendency to focus on some near and often dear person. If the frustration continues and is not in some way relieved, the psychodynamism may proceed to resentment, anger, jealousy, hatred, vengeance, and rage. On the other hand, when the basic drives for food and sex are satisfied, there is usually muscular relaxation, calm repose, and a general good feeling of well-being and contentment—in short, satisfaction.

It thus becomes significant that the naturally operating ethical principle, which can be induced from the plethora of human experience, takes into account the basic biological factor of satisfaction, that amazing emotional and conditionable feeling associated with the fulfillment of the drives for food and sex.

There are then several important ethical theories regarding human purposes, motivation, and conduct. They range from the rather selfish hedonism to altruistic social idealism, from harmonious adaptation to environments to self-conscious and adjustable individualism, and from utilitarianism to pragmatism, and with the probability of a naturally operating ethical principle which derives from biologically built-in neural mechanisms associated with adaptive and survival factors. What is ordinarily called "medical ethics," which is really merely a matter of decent etiquette, has scarcely ever been concerned with any genuine ethical theory, although social idealism is usually professed by medical apologists, and frank hedonism is practiced by members of the profession.

Medical Applications of Ethical Theory

A distinction should wisely be kept in mind between normative ethical concepts on one hand, and descriptive ethical theory on the other. The former presumes authoritatively to decide what people ought or ought not to do, usually omitting reference to purposes, or merely assuming social welfare as the overriding purpose in living for us all. The latter attempts to describe what may actually motivate people with respect to purposes, goals, objectives, conditioning, and physiological and psychological factors in behavior. Descriptive ethics also takes into account the difference between mood and behavior; mood is an individual subjective matter, while behavior is viewed from the standpoint of the social milieu. It is difficult to estimate the extent to which mood and behavior may coincide in relation to ethical theory in any given individual. This is one of the major problems in practical psychiatry.

It is interesting to try to apply the various ethical theories, which have been considered, to current medical problems. With regard to organ transplantation, for instance, it is clear that recipients are primarily motivated by hedonistic principles, in the sense that they are concerned with individual survival, while the donors and their families are relying on the tenets of Platonic social idealism, and the members of the surgical team are chiefly activated by a practical pragmatism. Thus there is much conflict of ethical principle in the situation, and unfortunately most of it is merely on a semiconscious or partially recognized level. Under these circumstances, it would seem wise for the members of the health professions and services who are involved to discuss the matter carefully and in detail with the prospective recipient, the proposed donor (or the donor's responsible agent), their respective families, and their religious and legal advisers. It might also be wise for the members of the health team involved to be conversant with the psychologically conflicting ethical principles which may be operative, so that individual motivations can be detected, exposed, and discussed. It might also be wise for the members of the health team to do everything possible to promote and maintain harmonious and trusting interpersonal relations toward recipients, donors, families, and religious and legal advisers, no matter what the outcome of the transplantation endeavor may be. It is to be remembered that there is practically no stronger imperative psychologically than for us to justify a faith or trust that has been placed in us.

The organ transplantation situation is an example of the characteristic situational ethic which is now being so well discussed by Joseph Fletcher. The point is that the situation is certain to change. Absolute ethical principles can thus no longer prevail. The wise solution may well be to consider with the utmost care the decisions which have to be made in the particular situation. It is the consequences of actions which must be foreseen as fully as possible, in order to prevent undesired effects.

Of course, the situation in regard to organ transplantation may change. Even after a successful kidney transplant, now almost routine, the donor of the healthy kidney may regret the loss, especially if subsequent kidney disorder develops, and there may be some psychological disability merely as a result of knowing that one kidney is gone. When organs for transplanting are taken from persons who have recently died, or who are supposed to be dead, there may be the technical problem, often legal, of just when death did occur. Perhaps organ banks may be developed, similar to existing blood, corneal, and ear-ossicle banks. Artificial organs are technically possible and are under development. These may solve the moral problems now associated with organ transplants.

With regard to hemodialysis, the ethical situation is complicated by economic factors. It may well be that improved technical devices will make hemodialysis possible on a home-use basis with relatively little expense for equipment and upkeep. Community financial aid, however, may always be needed when indigent patients are involved. This expense could well become a continuing item in community budgets. Cutting such budgets under the guise of economy might be politically expedient and justified under an ethic of pragmatism. It would be morally reprehensible under either an ethic of hedonism or of social idealism. What indigent patient could be found in our sophisticated culture who would voluntarily forgo a lifesaving available procedure in order to save money for the community?

We still have some time in which to prepare ourselves for the broad moral problems that may arise when genetic control becomes possible through gene manipulation. The matter is already under consideration, and Bentley Glass raised the moral issues at the recent Genetics Congress in Japan. The big question will be, "Who will decide?" Can decisions on genetic manipulation be left to democratic procedure with legal and thus authoritative power to make decisions over individual cases, or will we have confidence enough in the responsible judgment of those who by training and experience may be qualified to make wise decisions for the future of our race? And who will be judge of their qualifications?

It is likely that legal difficulties surrounding artificial insemination will be resolved by appropriate court decisions. It may be necessary, however, to make many changes in many of our laws which have become archaic in the light of current scientific knowledge and reasonable opinion based thereon. The difficulty in changing laws is exemplified in the slowness with which long-outmoded laws on abortion can be changed. Here it is clearly demonstrable that the present restrictive laws do great individual and social harm, yet the machinery for change is rusty.

There is much discussion over "informed consent" on the part of patients to any procedure proposed to be used upon them. It should be remembered that even a contractual agreement signed by a patient giving presumed informed consent to an operation or other procedure is not binding if that patient sub-sequently brings suit for malpractice, or for recovery of alleged damage inflicted by a member of the health professions involved in the case. The lex talionis principle, an eye for an eye, as invoked by Hammurabi millennia ago, still operates.

Emphasizing the personal responsibility of physicians in medical practice, Fletcher says that a doctor owes patients the truth as fully and as honestly as owing skill and proper care, excepting only when a patient is so mentally ill as not to be able to understand. This responsibility goes further to the use of every aspect of tact and gentleness that can be used, with every care to avoid hastiness, casualness, or unpleasantness in the telling of the truth. A trustful patient deserves a compassionate physician, and a duty of every physician is honest exposition to patients in terminology suited to their intelligence.

Currently we are vigorously discussing informed consent in regard to undertaking experimental procedures of a biomedical nature. Here again it should be remembered that any consent given by a patient does not prevent that patient from bringing suit to recover alleged damage inflicted by a physician or member of the staff of a hospital. The consent may act as a deterrent to a patient from initiating a suit for alleged damages, but it may also operate as an intention to reduce the care and caution that doctors and hospital staff must always exercise toward every patient, whether the patient is undergoing diagnostic testing, treatment, or direct medical experimentation. By any ethical theory, even that of practical pragmatism, the obligation remains with the members of the health professions and their associates to do everything they can on behalf of their patients' welfare, sacrificing themselves where necessary in order to do so.

Every treatment or diagnostic procedure undertaken on any patient is an experiment in the sense that the outcome cannot be predicted with certainty. Treatment with drugs, with surgery, or with physical or mental manipulation cannot be affirmed as completely safe in every patient; nor is there any certainty that every diagnostic procedure is without possible harm. Every patient presents a new, unique, and different research problem to the members of the health professions who may be consulted and who may undertake diagnosis and treatment. The risks of treatment must always be estimated against the risks of the disease or injury. Patients should be informed of these risks and make the decisions themselves as to whether or not treatment should proceed. There is thus a moral obligation to take the consequences that may result from the decision, always assuming that care is taken to prevent harm. If treatment or diagnostic testing results in harm, civil suit is possible to recover alleged damages.

The matter of informed consent is stirring comment in relation to the study of new drugs. In our University of California Pharmacology Laboratory, we developed such drugs as vinyl ether for anesthesia, carbarsone for amebiasis, iodochlorhydroxyquin (Vioform) for intestinal infections, the amphetamines for nervous stimulation, and nalorphine as a morphine antagonist. In doing this, we followed the rule that those of us who were interested in the drugs we were studying would be the first to take them ourselves, after animal experiments had indicated the character of biological activity and the extent of toxicity on single or repeated administration. It was only after we were convinced of the relative safety and effectiveness of the new drug and tried it ourselves, that we would undertake its study in other human subjects. In my opinion, this is a sound way to proceed.

It was too hasty use of new drugs under commercial pressure that resulted in the abuses which have brought such a flood of crippling red tape which bureaucracy now imposes in the de-

velopment of new drugs. Perhaps here, the guiding ethical principle could well be Platonic social idealism, with reasonable
regard for individual rights and welfare. In any case, the naturally operative principle of adaptive satisfaction would probably
be involved.

In Prospect

The moral problems arising from modern biomedical progress are not the exclusive responsibility of biomedical scientists
nor of members of the health professions or services. They are
the collective responsibility of all intelligent people and may
require extensive social discussion before socially acceptable
solutions may be agreed upon. A basic responsibility of biomedical scientists and of members of the health professions and
services is to place before the public all the verifiable information
incident to biomedical advance in condensed and readily understandable language. It may then be possible, with recognition of
the various ethical principles involved, to get the public understanding and support that will help us to use our technical tri-
umphs in worthy ways for individual and social welfare.

MEDICAL ETHICS AND
MORALS IN A NEW AGE

Paul S. Rhoads, M.D.

The principles of medical ethics have been enunciated through the ages: in the Babylonian code of Hammurabi, 2,000 B.C.; in the writing of Charoka and Susruta—Hindu writers of known antiquity; in the writing of Hippocrates; in the teachings of Christ and his disciples; in the writing of Maimonides; and, in modern times, in the Code of Percival in 1803.

The physician always sees himself as one who, because of his peculiar relationship with those he serves, has special responsibility: to be competent, to be honest, to hold a patient's life as a sacred trust. Hippocrates said, "A physician should be an upright man, instructed in the art of healing . . . modest, sober, patient, prompt to do his whole duty without anxiety; pious without going so far as superstition, conducting himself with propriety in his profession and in all the actions of his life." [1]

Christ said it for all doctors and all men more succinctly: "Therefore all things whatsoever ye would that men should do to you, do ye even so to them: for this is the law and the prophets" (Matt. 7:12, K.J.V.).

No matter how far we may fall short of the ideals we set for our profession, all of us will agree that our members have always strived and must continue to strive to be good men as well as good physicians. It is significant, I think, that at the first real meeting of the American Medical Association, in 1847, the two principal items of business were the establishment of a code of ethics and the creation of minimal requirements for medical education. It was not until 1955 that a serious attempt was made to separate the tenets of medical etiquette from the principles of medical ethics, a distinction which was so clearly described by Leake in his introductory essays to the compilation of Percival's writings.[2] Noteworthy, too, is the fact that in the preamble to the sharply condensed "Principles of Medical Ethics," published by the AMA in 1958, the importance of any "code" to control the actions of physicians in a bewildering variety of situations calling for compassion, clear thinking, and good judgment is acknowledged. The preamble to the 1966 version states:

"These principles are intended to aid physicians individually and collectively in maintaining a high level of ethical conduct. They are not laws but standards by which a physician may determine the propriety of his conduct in his relationship with patients, with colleagues, with members of allied professions, and with the public." [3]

The guidelines are there, and volumes have been and are being written about their application to individual problems. The amplifications and the rules of professional etiquette are well worth our study. In the end, however, the countless decisions each of us makes day by day on the basis of his individual convictions of right and wrong will determine whether our collective conscience works for the ultimate good of those we serve. How this conscience is to be kept sensitive and dominant and true in a time when so many influences are present to dull it, is one of the urgent problems of the day.

Perhaps I am naïve, but I do not believe that standards of conduct in our relationship with patients and with our fellow practitioners have seriously deteriorated yet in our profession—this in spite of the fact that precious little is said about it in our medical schools. The high standards set by our medical forebears in the privacy of their consulting rooms, in the homes which they visited, and in their research laboratories seem to have had their effect. Patients have been taught to place their confidence in us, and even our younger men—for the most part—do not seem to betray their trust. Whether this state of affairs will continue under modern conditions will depend upon how clearly we see the problem and what we shall do about it. Curricula are already overcrowded, but the ethical considerations of a patient's relationship with his doctor are of sufficient importance to warrant thoughtful discussions of these matters with every medical student in every medical school.

Let us turn now to some of the special problems of medical ethics and morals.

The Patient's Fees

I was disturbed to learn from the chairman of the Committee on Professional Fees of the Chicago Institute of Medicine that fee splitting, although prohibited by local and state societies and hospital staffs, is still practiced in Illinois and presumably in most other states of the nation. The committee has recommended state legislation to declare the practice unlawful and provide proper penalities. Although many physicians believe that this abuse cannot be stopped by legislation, putting a statute on the books can, at least, prevent greedy physicians from deducting fees paid to other physicians for referral as legitimate expenses of practice.

Although it is unlikely that any one of us would openly condone fee splitting, there are subtler forms of improperly burdening the patient with costs for medical services. For instance, when in hospital practice it becomes necessary for a patient to have the services of three to five physicians, is an effort made to see to it that the total charge for professional services is not exorbitant? All of the physicians concerned may piously observe that they have no control over the fees of the other specialists; however, they do have control of their own. Are they careful to see that the patient is not overcharged? Do we or do we not yield to the temptation to pad a bill a little because Medicare or some private insurance carrier is paying a substantial part of it?

Hospital costs are by no means the sole concern of the attending physicians, but they surely share in this responsibility. Current estimates of the average per diem cost of hospitalization per patient are approximately fifty-eight dollars. Furthermore, the yearly increase of 15 percent in daily cost which now obtains is apt to continue through the remainder of this decade. The bulk of this increase is from added cost of manpower services compounded from several sources. It apparently requires an average of 2.7 persons on the hospital payroll to take care of patients who seemed to be fairly well-cared-for when the ratio was about half what it is now. Furthermore, these people have much higher pay scales. Medicare, by requiring that each physician who was formerly an employee of the hospital render a separate bill, has increased the overhead charges of such physicians and thus put a further burden on the patient. Also, the major reallocation of hospital charges, undertaken because of the Medicare stipulation that laboratory services be billed at cost, have required hospital administrators, in order to maintain hospital solvency, to commensurately increase bed costs to an unheard-of level. This has worked to the distinct disadvantage of patients not receiving Medicare benefits. The sins that are committed in the name of cost-accounting to determine what should be fair service charges may not all be willful, but they are hard on the patient's pocketbook. To add to all this, attending physicians and house staff are often inexcusably prodigal and careless in ordering expensive procedures when they are not really necessary. For instance, a brain scan at one hospital costs the patient one hundred and four dollars. There are times when it may be of critical importance in making a diagnosis, but if Blue Cross or the government were not paying the bill, most of these and other unduly costly tests often would and could properly be avoided.

Why are these considerations brought up in a discussion of medical ethics? It is because to be a party to anything which is not to the best interest of our patients is unethical. It is difficult to subordinate group self-interest to the welfare of the patient when individual responsibility is not pinpointed. Unless hospital administrators, physicians, insurance carriers, and government officials get together and unselfishly attack the urgent problem of dangerously escalating medical costs, the public will take the matter into its own hands. We shall then have government controls which may be quite unpalatable to all of us.

The Incompetent or Irresponsible Physician

Some doctors, because of mental laziness or character disorders, should never have been allowed to graduate from medical schools. Others, because of lack of motivation, have not kept up with medical progress. Others have taken up questionable practices as well as continued their adherence to methods which are clearly outmoded. Hospital staffs and county medical societies have the mechanisms to enforce discipline among their members. They do this reasonably well, but not well enough. But what can be done with the incompetent, renegade physician who refuses to join medical societies and is content to carry on his questionable practice in his office, without hospital facilities? In 1965, only eighteen states had laws for disciplining such physicians; in many of these, the definitions of incompetence are so vague as to make prosecution very difficult.[4]

Milford O. Rouse, M.D., past president of the AMA, has urged that state boards of medical examiners be more aggressive in publicizing their availability to consider abuses and provide appropriate disciplinary measures. In states which do not have laws to handle such cases, the state boards and medical associations must seek legislation to curb unethical medical practices and revoke licenses of the offending physicians.

Abortion

Although there is no way of determining the actual number of illegal abortions in this country, it is estimated to be more than one million per year. About ten thousand pregnancies are terminated by licensed physicians in accredited hospitals with the knowledge and concurrence of consulting physicians.[5] There is great disparity in the beliefs of different religious faiths and those of individual physicians regarding the propriety of artificially terminating pregnancy. However, modern medical discoveries, particularly the recognition of prenatal influences which make it extremely likely that a physically or mentally handicapped child will be born, have made it imperative that the matter of therapeutic abortion be restudied. It is obvious that

almost all the existing state laws regarding abortion are outmoded. In forty-five states, the laws have permitted induced
termination of the pregnancy only to save the life of the mother.
In the remaining five states and the District of Columbia, the
added indication of protecting the health or safety of the mother
is recognized.[6] Changes in the law to implement the Model Penal
Code recommended by the American Bar Association in consultation with the AMA have now been made in Colorado and North
Carolina. In twenty-one other states, bills to change the abortion
statutes have been introduced, or study commissions are at work
to that end.

A recent poll indicates that the majority of physicians support
the stand of the Reference Committee on Human Reproduction
of the AMA which was reported at the June 1967 meeting of the
House of Delegates. It is as follows:

> The American Medical Association is cognizant of the fact that
> there is no consensus among physicians regarding the medical in-
> dications for therapeutic abortion. However, the majority of physi-
> cians believe that, in the light of recent advances in scientific
> medical knowledge, there may be substantial medical evidence
> brought forth in the evaluation of an occasional obstetric patient
> which would warrant the institution of therapeutic abortion either
> to safeguard the health or life of the patient, or to prevent the
> birth of a severely crippled, deformed or abnormal infant.
>
> Under these special circumstances, it is consistent with the
> policy of the American Medical Association for a licensed physi-
> cian in a hospital accredited by the Joint Commission on Accred-
> itation of Hospitals, and in consultation with two other physicians
> chosen because of their recognized professional competence who
> have examined the patient and have concurred in writing, to be
> permitted to prescribe and administer treatment for his patient
> commensurate with sound medical judgment and currently estab-
> lished scientific knowledge. Prior to the institution of a therapeu-
> tic abortion, the patient and her family should be fully advised
> of the medical implications and the possible untoward emotional
> and physical sequelae of the procedure.
>
> In view of the above, and recognizing that there are many
> physicians who on moral or religious grounds oppose therapeutic
> abortion under any circumstances, the American Medical Associa-
> tion is opposed to induced abortion except when:

(1) There is documented medical evidence that continuance of the pregnancy may threaten the health or life of the mother, or

(2) There is documented medical evidence that the infant may be born with incapacitating physical deformity or mental deficiency, or

(3) There is documented medical evidence that continuance of a pregnancy, resulting from legally established statutory or forcible rape or incest may constitute a threat to the mental or physical health of the patient;

(4) Two other physicians chosen because of their recognized professional competence have examined the patient and have concurred in writing; and

(5) The procedure is performed in a hospital accredited by the Joint Commission on Accreditation of Hospitals.

It is to be considered consistent with the principles of ethics of the American Medical Association for physicians to provide medical information to State Legislatures in their consideration of revision and/or the development of new legislation regarding therapeutic abortion.[7]

The jurists who helped shape this model code are well-aware that liberalization of the statute in no way frees the individual physician from making value judgments in every case based on his own concepts of right and wrong. Doctors will disagree on what constitutes a hazard to the health of the mothers. Few will argue that rubella (German measles) contracted by the mother in the second or third months of pregnancy constitutes a very definite risk to the integrity of the unborn child. But the possible hazard to the fetus from the use of such drugs as the phenothiazines; methotrexate; cortisone and its analogues; heroin; chloroquine and its derivatives; and many others is more debatable.

Criminal abortion is a very old problem. American medicine's stand on it is unequivocal and well-understood. We should be unyielding in our condemnation of it, and more aggressive in our prosecution of professional abortionists. Better definition of the authorized grounds for therapeutic abortion should make this possible.

Euthanasia

Even the term "euthanasia" bothers us. If we take it to mean putting a person to death painlessly even if he has an incurable and painful disease, our sensibilities are shocked. Yet if we include in our concept the failure to use all modern devices to maintain life a little longer—as we must—we are faced with a dilemma which all of us long frequently to avoid. Here, if ever, the physician must make some value decisions which are his alone and which he must make in his heart of hearts.

Our colleagues, the lawyers and the clergymen, are giving the matter serious thought. They would like to help us, but they cannot make the decisions. George P. Fletcher, J.D. of the Law School of Boston College, makes the following conclusion in a scholarly discussion of the problem:

> It will not do for the medical profession to demand that we lawyers devise a legal definition of death. There might be many uses of a legal definition of death; one might wish to know the time of death to apply rules on the disposition of the decedent's estate. But this is not what medical practitioners have in mind. It seems that they should like to have a clear standard for deciding when and when not to render aid to their dying patients. Sweden's Dr. Crafoord has proposed that a patient be declared legally dead when his EEG reading is flat. The standard is clear and easy to apply, but it is morally insensitive. Should one totally disregard all the other factors: the likelihood of recovery, the family's financial position, the patient's expressed wishes, other demands on hospital facilities, and the attending physician's time? Even if we could formulate a just resolution of these conflicting factors today, would it be a resolution that would remain fair in the face of medical innovation? It surely would not. What one regards as excessive and extraordinary today might well become commonplace in a few years. A legal standard of death, which would define the limits of the doctor's duty to his patient, would be an overly rigid solution to a problem that changes dimensions with each medical innovation.[8]

In the same symposium in which Professor Fletcher gave the legal view, the Very Reverend Brian Whitlow, Dean of the Anglican Christ Church Cathedral, Victoria, British Columbia, finished with the following statement:

In my view, essential medical or nursing care must always be given: food, warmth, washing, and easing of bodily position. But beyond that, decisions must be left to the physician. Medical opinion must always be the basis for deciding whether there is any reasonable hope of recovery.

An underlying principle of Christianity is that the love of God and of one's neighbors must be given priority at all times. Christ respected the Ten Commandments and the other traditional laws but gave this principle a priority over them all. I believe that the Christian position in the end comes to this: if the doctor is sincerely and selflessly trying to do the best for his patient, he is more likely to take the right course than if we try to draw up hard-and-fast rules to guide him in all cases.[9]

The development of mechanical devices such as the defibrillator, the artificial respirator, the heart stimulator, the bypass device to aerate blood during open-heart surgery, the artificial kidney, organ transplants, and other innovations have forced physicians to try to define the actual limit of a human life and to make difficult decisions as to whether—with the use of measures such as those just mentioned—they are prolonging life or prolonging the act of dying. When dealing with a comatose aged patient who has had a cerebrovascular accident and in whom there is no hope of restoring any useful or happy existence, few doctors have any qualms in withholding antibiotics and extraordinary mechanical means to prolong life. In such instances, the family should be consulted, the situation discussed with nurses and house staff, and note of the course decided upon made in the patient's chart.

In the case of younger persons in which the apparent death has been sudden, as from bacterial or allergic shock, anesthesia accidents, asphyxia (as, for example, a child shut in a refrigerator) and the like, there is little question that all efforts to restore respiration and heart function must be made. When to stop such resuscitative efforts depends upon one's own assessment of criteria such as: (1) fixed, dilated pupils; (2) complete absence of reflexes to painful stimuli; (3) complete absence of respiration and heartbeat for five minutes after respiration has stopped; and (4) a flat electroencephalogram curve. Such evaluation of evidence becomes of critical importance when the use of cadaver organs is being planned for a renal or heart transplant, for the chances of a good result depend, in a large measure, on getting the organ to be transplanted at the earliest possible moment after the patient is declared dead. There was much soul-searching on this point among the participants in the Ciba Foundation symposium on ethics in medical progress.[10] Someone must have the moral courage to make decisions when to use extraordinary measures to prolong life and when to stop them. No rigid rules can be laid down. Every physician must, in these circumstances, do what his deepest conscience dictates.

Human Experimentation

There is no sidestepping the fact that procedures which cannot be truthfully called anything but experimental have, through the ages, been done on human beings. Many times, patients have been unwilling subjects of medical experiments, and sometimes harm has come to them as a result. Experiments done without the patient's knowledge and consent cannot be condoned even on the grounds that they contributed to the ultimate good of mankind. As medical practice becomes the concern of the whole community, will the individual patient's welfare be as profound a responsibility to medical researchers as in the past? I think it will. But new safeguards which regulate human experimentation are being proposed.

The Declaration of Helsinki containing recommendations for the guidance of doctors in clinical research was adopted by the World Medical Association in 1964. Its basic principles are as follows:

1. Clinical research must conform to the moral and scientific principles that justify medical research, and should be based on laboratory and animal experiments or other scientifically established facts.
2. Clinical research should be conducted only by scientifically qualified persons and under the supervision of a qualified medical man.
3. Clinical research cannot legitimately be carried out unless the

importance of the objective is in proportion to the inherent risk to the subject.

4. Every clinical research project should be preceded by careful assessment of inherent risks in comparison to foreseeable benefits to the subject or to others.

5. Special caution should be exercised by the doctor in performing clinical research in which the personality of the subject is liable to be altered by drugs or experimental procedure.[11]

In elaboration of the principles, it is stipulated that non-therapeutic research on human beings must never be undertaken without their informed consent, but that, regardless of consent, responsibility for the procedure always remains with the medical investigator. In research combined with professional care, use of the therapeutic measure under investigation is justified in the acquisition of new knowledge only if it promises therapeutic value for the patient.

In the Ciba Foundation symposium on medical ethics, the question of coercion of donors of organs was brought up repeatedly. Starzl made the point that every effort was made to inform prisoners who were prospective donors of healthy kidneys that there would be no recompense to them in the way of financial reward or reduction of period of servitude. Only 2 percent of four thousand prisoners responded to the appeal for volunteers. Starzl hoped that the motivation of each prisoner donor was that he might be in a position "to contribute to his return to society." [12]

Daube, a British jurist, took issue with the use of prisoners for any medical experiment, insisting that absolutely no coercion should be exercised against a prospective donor. He flatly ruled out all prisoners and children as donors since they were not completely free to make decisions for themselves. The age of consent, he argued logically, should be the age allowable for military conscription.

The position of physicians in the matter of human experimentation is summed up well in an editorial in the *New England Journal of Medicine:* "The principles involved are, in substance, that the subject of an experiment involving any risk must stand to benefit by it; that his informed consent must be obtained to the fullest degree possible; finally and more important than any specific rules that have yet been devised, the investigator must be 'intelligent, informed, conscientious, compassionate, responsible.' " [13]

Medical Secrecy

The following statement appears in the "Principles of Medical Ethics" of the AMA: "A physician may not reveal the confidences entrusted to him in the course of medical attendance, or the deficiencies he may observe in the character of patients, unless he is required to do so by law or unless it becomes necessary in order to protect the welfare of the individual or of the community." [14]

How we are to keep careful records of our patients and still follow the spirit of the rule just stated, I do not know. The house staff, nurses, attending physicians, and consultants are allowed free access to patients' records in the hospital. Many other persons in the hospital gain such access, whether it is allowed or not. It seems to be easy for physicians' office records to become public property also. If a patient is involved in a traffic accident which subsequently becomes the subject of a legal controversy over personal injury, defense lawyers have the opportunity to examine his entire office record, even though the bulk of it contains confidential material totally unrelated to the accident. I have tried to resist such intrusion into what I considered purely private records but have been ordered to send the entire record to the lawyer for perusal and copying. Beyond this, reports to insurance companies, social security officers, and the like, intrude into the sanctity of private communication. I know of no way to combat this trend except to avoid as much as is practicable entering on the record those things which may be detrimental to the patient's welfare if revealed. This, of course, is not always possible and it is sometimes dishonest. All we can do—for instance, in revealing to a prospective employer facts which may compromise a patient's chance of obtaining a job—is to let the patient know what we are doing, then be as truthful as we can.

Comment

One could go on with endless problems confronting the modern physician which involve sensitive perception and judgment in acting for the best interests of the patient and for those of his family and community as well. In the end all one can say —as has been said before—is that the guidelines have been set forth in the many good statements of principles of medical ethics available to all of us. As I see it, each of us, using these principles as a standard by which to judge his own conduct and decisions, must obey the dictates of his own conscience. We are, without question, entering a new era in which the long-established, sacred, and very personal relationship between patient and doctor is in jeopardy. Modern medicine is broadly based, with a variety of specialists, professional and nonprofessional, cooperating in the care of a single patient. In many instances, an outside agency pays the bill. How, in this complex relationship, we are to preserve and be worthy of the trust of our patients who almost literally place their lives in our hands should be a matter of deep concern to all of us.

I have confidence in the young men entering our profession. One cannot work with them long without finding much of the idealism and devotion which we think characterized the generation of doctors before them. But, confronted with the kinds of problems considered in this communication, they will have some hard thinking and soul-searching to do. The new direction in which American medicine is going is not necessarily bad because it is different. William Osler wisely said, "The philosophies of one age have become the absurdities of the next, and the foolishness of yesterday has become the wisdom of tomorrow." [15]

But the problems will not solve themselves. Amid our preoccupations with deoxyribonucleic acid and ribonucleic acid, and the wonders revealed by the electron microscope, it is time we made a place in our curricula for brief consideration of the deeper issues upon which human health and happiness depend. Do our young men see human ills merely as thrilling challenges to scientific achievement? Or do they see their patients as fellow children of God who need their sympathetic understanding and encouragement? People will continue to get sick at home and will need to be cared for at home, and at all hours of the day and night. Will our young doctors be willing to give them the devoted service that they need? Is the modern physician equipped to be helpful in matters of marital dissension, in the serious problems of teen-agers, in the heartaches that result from alcoholism and drug addiction, in the sensitive situation of a patient facing certain death from cancer? Does he have the moral stamina to admit mistakes that have been injurious to his patients? If he feels that all of these problems that try men's souls are concerns only of the psychiatrist or the clergyman, he is far from being a complete physician. Personally, I think the step taken by the AMA in creating the Committee on Medicine and Religion is very pertinent to today's problems. It is time we had some counsel from our colleagues among the clergy and in the fields of philosophy and sociology. With their help, we should be able better to focus our attention on the needs of the whole man—mental and spiritual as well as physical. Fortunately, physicians are beginning to wrestle with these questions in a serious way.

I close with the exhortation penned by Sir Thomas Browne, the young London physician who, more than two centuries ago, gave us his timeless *Religio Medici* and *Christian Morals:* "Live by the old ethics and the classical rules of honesty. Put no new names or notions upon authentic virtues or vices. Think not that morality is ambulatory; that vices in one age are not vices in another; or that virtues which are under the everlasting seal of right reason, may be stumped by opinion. And therefore, though vicious times invent the opinion of things, and set up new ethics against virtue, yet hold onto the old morality; and rather than follow the multitude to do evil, stand like Pompey's Pillar conspicuous by thyself and single in integrity." [16]

ETHICAL AND LEGAL QUESTIONS POSED BY RECENT ADVANCES IN MEDICINE

James Z. Appel, M.D.

The tense and highly emotional drama that has been presented to the public by the various media of mass communication recently in the form of an almost blow by blow description of five human heart transplant operations has brought sharply into focus the legal and ethical problems with which the medical profession has been wrestling for quite a few years. While there was avid attention paid to the publicity about the experiments in Houston with a mechanical heart and its application to the human body as a partial substitute for the human heart, these experiments did not stimulate in the public's mind the ethical and legal complexities that are presently receiving much thought from various segments of society. The development of the mechanical kidney, the successful replacement of a faulty valve in a man's heart with a valve from a pig's heart in Great Britain and one from a calf's heart in India, the successful excision of dead heart muscle in patients after coronary occlusion, the maintenance of life of a heart attack victim through a lengthy operation in Canada, the more than two thousand successful human kidney transplantations that have taken place, and the less successful and smaller number of human liver transplantations attracted much less attention from the public than did the human heart transplantations.

It is difficult to say why this has occurred. Perhaps it was the fact that the new heart, a new heart for an old worn-out heart, was involved. Perhaps it was because the heart transplant operation presented a situation which was inevitable and not present in the other types of human to human transplantation, except for liver transplant, and that is that the donor must die. Liver transplantations have been too few to have attracted much attention. Nevertheless, here too someone must die. Perhaps the symbolic significance of the heart as the site of life and the source of love and all the emotions intensified the impact. Who knows? Certainly kidney transplants would not create the same feelings since the donor does not have to die, can live, and does live. Such gifts to a fellow being have been considered the height of generosity. But in the case of the heart, are these scientists moving too far and too fast in their zeal for new knowledge and for fame? Has the technique been developed to such an extent so that a scientist has the right to extend hope for a better existence following the operation? Might not the over-enthusiastic heart surgeon be tempted to declare the donor dead before death occurred in order to have a viable heart to transplant? If the surgery proves successful, will there not be a demand for secondhand hearts which will far outstrip the supply? How will priorities for eligibility as a recipient be established and who will make these decisions? Is the total procedure ethical? Is it legal? As we develop the ability and skill to transplant organs and as multiple organ transplants are performed on one individual, perhaps even the brain, in the not too far distant future, may be transplanted. Then one may inquire "Who is that body that is housing many spare parts donated by many different donors?"

A scientific achievement in medicine occurred recently which may be of much more significance than organ transplantation. This is the creation of life itself by a group of scientists at Stanford University. They were able to produce synthetically living deoxyribonucleic acid. What type of ethical problems might the exploitation of this achievement present? Will we be able to create a virus that will prevent cancer, mental disease, or the rejection of organ transplants? Will this be a means to control quality in future generations as we control quality in animals by selective breeding? Do we want this power over future mankind?

I have posed many questions. There are, I am sure, others that you will think of. I do not have the answers but I can elaborate and offer suggestions. Since death is inevitable for the donor of a heart or a liver, it is essential that we understand what death is and be able to identify when it occurs rather precisely. Biologically speaking there is no "moment of death." Legally and from a religious point of view there *is* such a moment. In these disciplines death is defined as the irreversible cessation of heart action or respiratory activity or both. But biologically death of a human being or animal is a process which might extend over as much time as several weeks since we know that the growth of hair and nails has continued that long after a person has been declared dead.

If we turn to the dictionary for a definition of death we find the prime definition as "the cessation of life; that state of being, animal or vegetable, in which all vital functions cease permanently." In the same dictionary we find that "vital functions" are "functions immediately necessary to life as those of the brain, heart, lungs, etc."

With the development of the sophisticated instruments we use today to restore the heartbeat in patients with cardiac arrest, ventricular fibrillation, and other forms of heart stoppage, physicians have already been questioning the use of heart stoppage and cessation of respiration as the legal sign of death. Successful restoration of independent heart action has often occurred several minutes after it has ceased beating. Many productive lives have been preserved. Some "vegetables" have been created. This poses grave consideration as to what kind of a person we will have if we institute and persist in cardiac resuscitation. Thus the physician might and usually does in such situations have to make several on-the-spot decisions. Should an attempt to restore heart action be made on all people who suffer such heart stoppage? Should the duration of the heart stoppage before applying heroic measures that might start it and restore independent action be considered in order to avoid producing a living body without a thinking brain? How long should efforts be maintained to convert an inactive heart to one that beats spontaneously? Physicians dread feeling responsible for producing a "vegetable" existence for the patient. Leaving emotions out of it, it is a matter of record that physicians have been successfully sued in courts of law for doing just this. They have also been successfully sued for failing to attempt to restore life to a patient whose heart has ceased beating.

Let us return to the consideration of the dying donor with an organ potentially to transplant. Should the physician attempt to restore heart action in the donor patient and then after a period of time turn off the resuscitator? If the heart does not continue to beat independently of the machine, should he declare the patient dead and then start the machine again so that there will be some circulation in the organ to be transplanted?

These questions have caused the medical scientist and the medical practitioner to wonder if we should not have new criteria to determine legal death. Since we have developed techniques to restore heart action, spontaneous heart action, long after mental activity of the brain has irreversibly ceased, perhaps the death of the brain should be the legal sign of death. Life in the brain can be determined by use of the electroencephalogram, the state of the pupils of the eyes, and other neurological signs. Incidentally, more and more hospitals are placing electroencephalograph machines in their emergency departments and their intensive care units or making such machines a part of the equipment that responds to the "code blue" emergency call.

These questions are being discussed throughout the entire medical world. The criteria for determination when death has occurred that have received acceptance by many physicians in most countries are the following:

1. Complete bilateral dilatation of the pupils with no reaction to local constricting stimuli.
2. Complete abolition of reflexes.
3. Complete cessation of respiration five minutes after cessation of mechanical respiration.

4. Falling blood pressure (maintenance of blood pressure demands increasing vasoconstrictor drugs).
5. Flat electroencephalogram.

The essential point is that if brain function is abolished and spontaneous circulation and respiration have ceased, the patient should be considered dead. Of equal importance, the determination that these criteria have been met should be made by the medical team which is in charge of the dying donor patient, never by the medical team responsible for the recipient patient.

Another question that presents itself is, "Who has the right to give permission for the removal of the organ after death?" Only a few religions have tenets opposing such removal or consider it immoral mutilation of the body. The Catholic Church has taken a definite position that the removal of an organ or organs from a deceased person is permissible for scientific purposes. It has questioned the prematurity of the recent heart transplant operations. But the English common law, the basis upon which many of our court decisions are rendered, declares that there are no property rights in the body of a dead person. This has been interpreted to mean that it is questionable if a person can will his or her body or any part of it to science. Common law does decree that there is a right of possession of the body which rests in the next of kin, but this is for burial purposes only.

While courts are not too often asked to act on these questions, sufficient legal activity has occurred so that legislation has been enacted in some states specifically permitting the willing of the cornea to eye banks and the body to science. Where such legislation exists it has been argued that if one may will the entire body to science one may will a part, such as an organ, to science to be used for transplantation purposes. Thirty-one of the states have some type of legislation on these matters but they differ widely in many respects. In all the state laws specific permission in writing must be obtained from the next of kin unless the donor himself has the legal right to will his body or organs. Permission of the next of kin may be difficult to obtain immediately following a fatal accident. Securing evidence that a proper will has been made likewise takes time, especially when the death occurs away from the home of the deceased. Time between death and transplantation is a very important factor so far as the success of the procedure is concerned.

In a similar vein, consent must be obtained from the recipient in an organ transplant procedure. Such consent must be an "informed consent." This means that the patient (the recipient) completely understands the procedure proposed, its potential benefits, and its possible adverse effects. He must understand fully the present condition as it exists without transplantation and what he might expect if no surgery is performed. The recipient must know that while he is living a most precarious life and has exhausted the traditional methods of treating the condition, if he undergoes a heart transplant he will die very promptly if it fails. He must understand that if it is only partially successful he might live but his life might be worse than it has been because of lack of knowledge and ability to overcome the rejection process.

The physician in charge of the recipient patient must be in a position of certainty in advising the patient that no other procedure or treatment is available to prevent his imminent death. There are inadequate guidelines for the physician to follow in reaching this decision other than qualified professional consultations. Even with such consultants to advise him, the physician is on his own and can only use his best judgment.

What guidelines we have to protect the patient and the physician were developed during the Nuremberg Trials following World War II when the world was appalled by the irresponsible human experimentation practiced by Nazi physicians. Based on the principles used during these trials, the World Medical Association adopted the so-called Helsinki Agreement, which has been adopted by most nation members of the United Nations and most national medical societies of the free nations.

It is difficult for the patient to make an objective appraisal of the information provided him and upon which he must make a literally vital decision. His primary desire is to get well, and if this is impossible, at least to get better. To accomplish this he is moved to accept any suggestions that seem the least bit encouraging. In spite of all the pros and cons presented by his physician and in spite of every effort the physician puts forth to explain the procedure and possible consequences in language that the patient might understand, the mental processes are driven by the desire to get well. The patient cannot completely understand the alternatives to a successful procedure or put proper weight upon them. The patient trusts his physician who sincerely believes the transplant is the one and only way to a cure but who might be just a bit prejudiced. Therefore, it is my opinion that the closest relatives should be drawn into the decision-making process. I realize their ability to make a decision or help the patient come to a decision is just as much handicapped by lack of understanding and by personal emotions. At least it is an added safeguard.

Regardless of how successful we become in the transplantation of human organs, the conquering of the rejection process, and all the complications that attend this procedure, we may never have available sufficient donor organs to meet the demand. Today only the worst possible risks are accepted as recipients for heart transplantations. As the technique improves, and I am sure it will, the strict medical indications for organ transplantation will be lessened so that more and more patients will be considered eligible. Undoubtedly organ source information centers will be established, as has already been done in Los Angeles, and more people will be willing to donate their organs after death. Certainly we will find a way to establish organ banks just as we do have eye banks and blood banks. In spite of all this, the demand will far exceed the supply.

We have this problem today in the hemodialysis of our patients with renal failure. There are many more patients in need of this kind of treatment than there are kidney machines to serve them. When this situation occurs, how will the decision be made and who will make the decision as to who shall receive a transplant, be accepted for dialysis, and live, and who shall be rejected and condemned to an early death? Shall such decisions be based on the general health of the recipient, his moral character, his family responsibility, his value to the community, or his wealth? The cost to maintain life on a kidney machine amounts to between $10,000 and $20,000 a year. A kidney transplant operation costs about $5,000, involves between fifteen and thirty scientists, physicians, technologists, and a considerable number of backup and substitute personnel, and, thereafter, costs about $1,000 a year to combat rejection. Shall only the wealthy receive a secondhand kidney, liver, or heart? On a recent date in Los Angeles there were eighty patients waiting for secondhand kidneys and only four were available.

In one of the oldest hemodialysis laboratories in this country, there are many potential beneficiaries of the machine who have to be rejected. As I understand the procedure followed in that laboratory, an anonymous committee of lay people who live in the area make the decisions with physicians used primarily as consultants. They take into consideration many things about the patient such as his general health, his morality, his social and family responsibilities, the part he plays in community life and its economy, and many others. Tenure on the committee is relatively short because it is recognized that such decision making has an awesome effect on the person asked to do so. But this is a job that has to be done and will have to be done more frequently in the future. Who will do it and on what basis will it be done?

During a television interview in New York, Dr. Barnard of Capetown, South Africa, who performed the heart transplant, was asked his views on the morality of his actions; he said: "My duty as a doctor is to treat the patient. As far as the donor was concerned I could not treat her anymore. She was beyond the stage when I had any medical knowledge or any know-how to treat her. So there my duty ended. As far as the recipient or the patient was concerned, I had only one way of treating him and that was to transplant a heart. And this was the treatment I gave this patient. I do not think this is immoral."

Neither do I. I do believe Dr. Barnard was fortunate that he could feel so sure of his premises. Perhaps it was an oversight and not a "Freudian slip" but I note that he referred to the donor as "the donor" and to the recipient as "the recipient or the patient." As was said before, I do not believe the same physician or medical team should pass judgment on the donor and the recipient. There probably were two teams in Capetown. Dr. Barnard did not make this point clear, and we must remember this was a short television interview.

The concern of society for answers to some of these questions has stimulated study groups of various sponsorship. The National Academy of Science developed criteria and guidelines which were very general but did call on a team of consultants. The Academy of Cardiology convened a symposium in Houston during which many and various opinions were expressed. The Congress of the United States received a bill introduced by Senator Mondale which would create a Commission on Health, Science, and Society consisting of fifteen members appointed by the President from among representatives of medicine, law, science, theology, philosophy, ethics, health administration, and government. Other organizations have also proposed investigative commissions on use of humans in medical research.

The proponents of such study groups are not only interested in developing legal, ethical, and moral questions which need solution but also are interested in the production of guidelines which will exercise some control on this type of research and those scientists who conduct such research. In establishing guidelines, the physician should resort to an old and proven safeguard included in the "Principles of Medical Ethics" of the American Medical Association, that involves the readiness to use consultants. Medicine has been divided into specialties and subspecialties. Often we decry this fragmentation. But here it serves a valuable purpose since it brings a variety of knowledge, interests, and approaches to a very serious problem. However, there should be no limitation to the medical profession for such consultants. Other disciplines should be involved, such as the legal profession, sociologists, the clergy, and others, as the circumstances demand. It should be remembered that in a democratic society such as the one in which we live, the complete freedom of any profession to regulate itself depends upon its doing so in a responsible manner. When, in the opinion of the people, it fails in exercising this responsibility, the people will demand and secure regulatory controls. To insure informed evaluation by the people, the people must be educated that the research is meeting the demands of society for scientific advancement, meanwhile protecting the rights and dignity of man.

I believe that organ transplants should continue. At present they should not be considered as an accepted form of treatment but as a form of research. Only teams of physicians and medical scientists who have demonstrated ability in the procedure gained from animal research and who have established a reputation for responsibility in the ethics of human experimentation should be permitted to carry out such research. The legal questions I have posed must, can, and will be solved. One more word about the legality of the procedure and that is, that where legal codes threaten such research, legislation should be passed that will permit it but at the same time will protect the donor, the recipient, and the medical team.

I believe great efforts should be made to solve the problems encountered in the transplantation of organs from animals to humans. Hearts from the calf and the pig lend themselves admirably for this purpose. Great efforts should be expended in furthering the development of miniaturized mechanical organ substitutes for human organs. We have far better prospects of being able to meet the demand by mass production of mechanical replacements than if we always rely on human organs for transplants. So far none of the mechanical substitutes approach the effectiveness of the human or animal transplants, at least until the rejection process takes place. Because the heart is a much simpler organ to reproduce mechanically than the highly specialized kidney or liver, perhaps most of our efforts in this research should be directed to mechanical hearts.

Continued and intensified effort should be directed toward learning how to prevent organ failure and how to recognize and medically correct an early failure in an organ. Success in this area may well obviate most organ transplantation operations.

Finally, somehow man must define or set a limit as to how far we should go in these efforts to prolong life. Even though we might be able to replace a worn-out brain some day, and I believe that is in the realm of future possibilities, we must accept the fact that some lives should not be prolonged. Certainly the medical profession is not qualified to make all these decisions by itself. Society must somehow become involved.

I have left you with many questions and few answers. At this time that is all that anyone can do. It is good that we recognize that there are questions and these questions must be answered before we go much further.

ETHICAL IMPLICATIONS OF
PROFESSIONAL COMPETENCY

There has been a great deal of publicity in the lay press at various times about so-called incompetence of physicians in the United States. Most of these tirades have been written by obviously prejudiced and, indeed, often misinformed writers. It is probable, however, that this unfortunate publicity may result in adverse responses which could affect the relationship between physician and patient or the physician and the hospital chaplain. I recognize that the medical profession is doing a great deal in the form of postgraduate education, but I would appreciate your opinion of the fundamental aspects of professional competency regarding the ethical responsibilities of the physician. Does the physician's professional competency really enhance the cooperation between physician and clergyman?

RESPONDENT: *Adolph R. Berger, M.D.*

The physician cannot and must not be the spiritual counselor for the patient. Yet the physician, by professional competency and humility, often can direct the patient (if he or she has not already done this spontaneously) to spiritual matters.

Fundamentally, the patient poses two questions to the physician: what is wrong with me? what can you, the physician, do about this illness? The questions sometimes go unanswered, either completely or in part, because of basic deficiencies in medical knowledge. However, given a patient whose illness is one for which effective diagnostic and therapeutic measures exist, the limiting factor then becomes the knowledge and resourcefulness, the competency, of the physician in his profession. That physicians vary in their abilities is self-evident. That physicians have been trying to remain abreast of the advances in their profession is seen in certification by specialty boards, attendance at hospital staff meetings or postgraduate courses, and other educational efforts. If the patient is assured of the professional adequacy—hopefully, superiority—of his doctor, he should have confidence that all of medicine's advances and advantages are known to his medical attendants (the collective term is used because consultants may be involved in the diagnosis or treatment of the illness at hand) and that the totality of medical knowledge can be employed for his welfare. The physician's suggestion, then, that the spiritual aspect of the patient's life be aided by the clergyman cannot be construed as a substitute for firm medical knowledge. Piety is no substitute for professional competency. Indeed, had not the patient been assured of that competency, he (or she) could suspect, probably correctly, that the piety was superficial, the worst sort of cover-up for professional ignorance.

Competency in medicine comes from several directions. In a spiritual sense, the physician must believe that whatever professional talents he possesses represent the free gifts of God, gifts like the gift of life, gifts with the implicit obligations that they be nurtured and used for the maximal benefit of patients. Could the physician, then, do less than strive for professional competency throughout the years of his practice? With this concept of competency, professional competency is one aspect of the physician's spiritual life which can be imparted to or sensed by the patient, and the physician becomes a more effective collaborator with the clergyman. Professional competency thus has clear and immediate relevance to the cooperative efforts of physician and clergyman.

Although the main emphasis in this question and its answer is on the role of the physician's professional competency in enhancing cooperation between physician and clergyman, the preamble to the question also contains one thought which cannot be allowed to go by without some comment. The idea has been raised that "unfortunate publicity may result in adverse responses which could affect the relationship" between the concerned parties.

Prejudiced and misinformed writers undoubtedly exist, and their writings, unhappily, may be published and even publicized widely. Sensational stories—whether about medical research, patient care, or professional competency—often really signify poor lines of communication. In the community at large, there is a great ignorance of medical facts, despite the educational campaigns of many national or local public health organizations. This general lack of medical knowledge and the insufficient exposure of the clergyman to medicine in his seminary or post-seminary years are understandable. The solution to the problem of "adverse reactions," though difficult at times, can be achieved in association with the various communications media. We in medicine must begin with the firm conviction that very few people really are trying to cause trouble. The lines of communication between the parties must be improved in order that fact may be distinguished from fiction. Above all, the lines must be two-way, and the messages transmitted in both directions must be sent and received in a spirit of true charity.

ETHICAL GUIDELINES FOR ORGAN TRANSPLANTATION

*It should be apparent that no stigma is attached to the perfor-
mance of human experiments per se; disgrace and infamy can
arise only through its misuse. The moral obligation of performing all human experiments, with due regard to the sensibility,
welfare, and safety of the subject, must not be violated. As
phrased by Claude Bernard in 1856, "Christian morals forbid
only one thing, doing ill to one's neighbor." So, among experiments that may be tried on man, those that can only do harm
are forbidden, those that are harmless are permissible, and those
that may do good are obligatory.*

RESPONDENT: *E. G. Shelley, M.D.*

The medical profession, in its never-ending search for ways
to save human life, relieve suffering, and improve health, has
always been motivated and guided by the principles expressed in
the above quotation. To achieve these goals, it has recognized
that proper standards must be established and followed in clinical investigation and experimentation involving human beings.

In 1946, the American Medical Association succinctly listed
three ethical guidelines to be followed in human experimentation in order to have such experimentation conform to medical
ethics: (1) voluntary consent must be obtained from the person
on whom the experiment is to be performed; (2) the dangers of
each experiment must have been previously investigated by animal experimentation; and (3) the experiment must be performed
under proper medical protection and management.

In 1964, the World Medical Association adopted the Declaration of Helsinki, which was later endorsed by the American Medical Association. The Declaration emphasizes "freely given consent" and differentiates between clinical research combined with professional care and nontherapeutic clinical research.

In 1966, the American Medical Association adopted a longer statement—"Ethical Guidelines for Clinical Investigation." In part, these guidelines state:

> In clinical investigation primarily for treatment,
> A. The physician must recognize that the physician-patient relationship exists and that he is expected to exercise his professional judgment and skill in the best interest of the patient.
> B. Voluntary consent must be obtained from the patient, or from his legally authorized representative if the patient lacks the capacity to consent, following: disclosure that the physician intends to use an investigational drug or experimental procedure; a reasonable explanation of the nature of the drug or procedure to be used, risks to be expected, and possible therapeutic benefits; an offer to answer any inquiries concerning the drug or procedure; and a disclosure of alternative drugs or procedures that may be available.

The "Principles of Medical Ethics" and these several statements have provided broad guidelines during the period when transplants of major body organs were first performed. In the opinion of the Judicial Council these principles continue to be valid.

Now, theologians, lawyers, and other public-spirited persons, as well as physicians, are discussing with deep concern the many new questions raised by the transplantation of vital organs. Man participates in these procedures: he is the patient in them; or he performs them. All mankind is the ultimate beneficiary of them.

A man, in the final analysis, must make a decision whether to permit or to perform a transplantation procedure. The decision must be a reasoned, intellectual decision, not an emotional decision. As medical science advances, and as technological skill increases, the ethical questions involved may become increasingly complex and difficult.

The Judicial Council, therefore, commends discussion of the moral, ethical, legal, social, and other aspects of clinical investigation, experimentation, and organ transplantation in human beings. It commends all efforts which encourage respect for the dignity of man, and which seek to sensitize man's ethical conscience.

The Judicial Council of the AMA offers the following statement for guidance of physicians as they seek to maintain the highest level of ethical conduct in their practices.

1. In all professional relationships between a physician and his patient, the physician's primary concern must be the health of his patient. He owes the patient his primary allegiance. This concern and allegiance must be preserved in all medical procedures, including those which involve the transplantation of an organ from one person to another where both donor and recipient are patients. Care must, therefore, be taken to protect the rights of both the donor and the recipient, and no physician may assume a responsibility in organ transplantation unless the rights of both donor and recipient are equally protected.

2. A prospective organ transplant offers no justification for relaxation of the usual standards of medical care. The physician should provide his patient, who may be a prospective organ donor, with that care usually given others being treated for a similar injury or disease.

3. When a vital, single organ is to be transplanted, the death of the donor shall have been determined by at least one physician other than the recipient's physician. Death shall be determined by the clinical judgment of the physician. In making this determination, the ethical physician will use all available, currently accepted scientific tests.

4. Full discussion of the proposed procedure with the donor and the recipient or their responsible relatives or representatives is mandatory. The physician should be objective in discussing the procedure, in disclosing known risks and possible hazards, and in advising of the alternative procedures available. The physician should not encourage expectations beyond those which the circumstances justify. The physician's interest in advancing scientific knowledge must always be secondary to his primary concern for the patient.

5. Transplant procedures of body organs should be undertaken (a) only by physicians who possess special medical knowledge and technical competence developed through special training, study, and laboratory experience and practice, and (b) in medi-

cal institutions with facilities adequate to protect the health and
well-being of the parties to the procedure.

6. Transplantation of body organs should be undertaken only after
   careful evaluation of the availability and effectiveness of other
   possible therapy.

7. Medicine recognizes that organ transplants are newsworthy and
   that the public is entitled to be correctly informed about them.
   Normally, a scientific report of the procedures should first be
   made to the medical profession for review and evaluation. When
   dramatic aspects of medical advances prevent adherence to accepted procedures, objective, factual, and discreet public reports
   to the communications media may be made by a properly authorized physician, but should be followed as soon as possible by
   full scientific reports to the profession.

In organ transplantation procedures, the right of privacy of
the parties to the procedures must be respected. Without their
authorization to disclose their identity the physician is limited
to an impersonal discussion of the procedure.

Reporting of medical and surgical procedures should always
be objective and factual. Such reporting will also preserve and
enhance the stature of the medical profession and its service to
mankind.

ETHICAL IMPLICATIONS OF
RENAL TRANSPLANTS

A ten-year-old boy has advanced renal disease. It has been suggested that his identical twin be the donor for a renal transplant operation. What are the social and ethical aspects of such organ transplants? Incidentally, the family is Catholic and I would appreciate the opinion of a priest as well as the judgment of a physician.

RESPONDENT: *Joseph E. Murray, M.D.*

Organ transplants, as a therapeutic maneuver to prolong life, are certainly justified as far as the recipient is concerned. Fifteen years have elapsed since the beginning of modern human experimentation in this field and at present, more than five hundred humans are living with transplanted kidneys. The original efforts were attempts to understand the medical, surgical, and immunological problems involved and could only have been worked out in humans. Had the problem remained a pure laboratory one, many pitfalls and problems peculiar to the human would never have been recognized and solved. For the prospective recipient, the only preoperative requirement is that all known methods of treatment have been tried and have failed.

The source of the kidney, however, provides a major moral, legal, and ethical problem. If the source is a recently deceased individual whose nearest relatives have voluntarily donated the kidney, there is no problem. If the source is an elective nephrectomy for the benefit of another human being, and a kidney is used which would otherwise be discarded, again, there is no problem. However, when the donor is a living healthy volunteer,

either a member or a nonmember of the family, a definite problem arises. Here we are embarking on a major surgical operation
with a slight, but definite, risk from anesthesia, operation, or
postoperative complications. This procedure is not for the benefit of the person being operated on, but for someone else. All
previous medical and surgical training has been geared to weigh-
ing the advantages and disadvantages in any one patient of a
proposed therapeutic measure. However, in this instance, for
the donor, a physiological deficit will always occur, and no possible good can accrue to him physically.

The volunteer kidney donor may, however, derive a certain
spiritual benefit from the act of donation, probably the purest
form of charity next to the giving of one's life. For a truly un-
pressured volunteer, this spiritual satisfaction can more than
compensate for the physical trial of a nephrectomy. The courts
in various states have recognized the validity of such a donation
in a minor child on the principle that the child would be harmed
psychologically, spiritually, and aesthetically if he were deprived
of the opportunity of donating a kidney to save his identical
twin.

Every voluntary operation to remove a kidney from a normal,
healthy human being must be weighed with great seriousness
and responsibility on the part of the participating physician
and surgeon.

RESPONDENT: *John J. Lynch, S.J.*

It should first be noted that on the question of organic transplantation inter vivos, the Roman Catholic Church has never
yet declared an official teaching. Consequently, in this matter
there is no authoritative doctrine to which a Roman Catholic
physician would be in conscience committed by virtue of his
allegiance to his church.

Private theologians, however, have been busily discussing
this problem ever since the question became a medical practi-
cality. Their professional (and fallible) opinions differ. Of those
who have expressed themselves publicly on the subject, the majority—it would seem safe to say—profess to see at least solidly

probable grounds for declaring this form of transplantation permissible under certain circumstances. A very articulate minority, however, can adduce reasons no less suasive for concluding to the contrary. This theological impasse is not likely to be resolved in the near future.

Those who challenge the permissibility of this form of organic transplantation do so because of a sincere conviction that only when it is necessary for one's own total medical good may one sacrifice a bodily member. In substantiation of this premise they are able to cite several papal statements which seem to concur with their position. And since the donor in a transplant transaction has physically only loss to show for his pains, this school of thought concludes—most logically, if their premise be granted—to a prohibition against the procedure.

Those who defend the licitness of the same procedure deny the exclusiveness of any principle which would allow bodily mutilation only for the total good of the patient himself. They maintain that the law of fraternal love—whereby one may do for another whatever one may legitimately do for self—can also be invoked in justification of certain organic transplants. Their reason, though weighty, are not altogether conclusive theologically; but neither are the contrary arguments submitted by the opposition.

Where does this theological deadlock leave the conscientious Roman Catholic physician? On the supposition that proper consent is obtained, it leaves him entirely free to follow in practice, if he so chooses, the opinion which grants him the greater liberty of medical action. No one is required to acknowledge as obligatory a prohibition which is at best objectively doubtful. In other words, no theologian could legitimately accuse of moral wrongdoing the physician who involves himself professionally in organic transplantation with due regard for those precautions which sound medical sense would prescribe for that procedure. Or to put it more positively, as one should, the doctor, who in medical prudence seeks to preserve human life by means of organic transplantation, can merit no less theologically than he does scientifically.

MEDICAL MISSIONARY SERVICE

I am a medical student giving serious consideration to service in the foreign field as a medical missionary. What special attributes and training would make me an acceptable candidate?

RESPONDENT: *Kenneth M. Scott, M.D.*

Whether you plan to become a short-term or a career medical missionary, you should have acquired professional knowledge and skills at least as good as the best available in the country to which you will go. The day has long passed when *any* medicine could be said to be better than no medicine at all. Prior experience in general practice or, better, full specialty training is a requisite for most service overseas. If you live in America, this means certification by an American specialty board, to be completed before going overseas or at least during the first furlough. This is important because of the increasingly prominent place that teaching has in most overseas medical institutions today.

Whether you serve in a developing country under a church mission board or under some secular agency, you will need utmost patience and tact and much humility. The worst thing a missionary can say is: "this is the way we do it in America." If you are married, your wife should be of one heart with you in this venture. Both of you must have a genuine love for people, as well as inner resources adequate for the day-to-day physical and emotional pressures you will experience.

Apart from professional excellence, the secret of being a good medical missionary has been described as "knowing God, knowing the people, and knowing the language." As to the latter, only a long-term career missionary is likely to know the people and their language. Since there is a basic difference in involvement between a career missionary doctor who has burned his bridges behind him and a "visiting fireman" who is here today and gone tomorrow, few mission boards will appoint and support a young doctor knowingly for only three or four years of missionary service, except under special circumstances.

If you are undecided about entering missionary service, try some short overseas service as a sampler. The Smith Kline & French fellowships awarded to selected medical students often provide excellent opportunities to observe missionary life and challenges. Or, when you have completed your medical training, you may wish to apply for some short-term service overseas by writing to the American Medical Association, the Christian Medical Society, Medicare, the Peace Corps, or to any of a large number of voluntary agencies, including your own church.

If you decide ultimately on a missionary vocation, you will discover that the contribution made by a career medical missionary often outweighs that made by government and other secular agencies having greater financial resources.

RESPONDENT: *Robert B. White, M.D.*

Three special attributes in my opinion should characterize a medical missionary candidate.

A love for people. Not all will look upon you as God's gift to their country or people. They will be in desperate need of help, but the sense of obligation to the help received and their own personal pride will often manifest itself by inexplicable actions of resentment—and you would probably do the same if you were in their position. Therefore, a very real love for the people and a manifest desire to understand their mores and culture are essential to your effectiveness and to the prevention of a personally destructive inner bitterness.

A love for learning. Opportunities for furthering your medical education while in missionary service will usually be limited. It is, therefore, essential that you develop disciplines for carrying on your own self-education by means of journals and up-to-date texts. But your love for medical knowledge is only half the

answer. Learning the language of the people is the only effective
way of communicating with them. Your appreciation of a people
and their culture will be greatly enhanced by understanding
and speaking their language.

A love for God. When the external props to one's faith are
cut asunder, the strength of the "inner man" is quickly revealed.
And the man whose love for and communication with God have
been established, through long practice of reflectiveness on life's
meaning and purpose, will be better able to cope when, as inevitably he must, he stands alone.

One final word: training depends very much on the type of
situation to which one will go. It is true that more and more the
demands in medical mission service are in the teaching field at
nursing or medical school level. Here, fully specialty training is
advisable, and in the field of public health, is especially needed.
If, however, one is to serve in a mission hospital in a relatively
primitive, direct-service situation, such specialization is not
necessary. Still, at least one year of residency, preferably surgical,
and a full course of tropical medicine are almost essential in most
of the developing areas of the world today.

SHOULD I GO TO MEDICAL SCHOOL?

Not infrequently I am asked by high school seniors and college undergraduates whether I would advise them, or indeed my own children, to study medicine as a career. If I understand the implications of their question, some of these bright and highly idealistic young men and women are searching for a profession which offers more than financial security or scientific achievement (in the sense of predominantly research activities). Would it not be reasonable and intellectually honest to describe medicine as an art rather than as a science? Can we not assure these students that a medical career is appropriate for them if they seek the warmth of human relations and the trust of patients gained by extending sympathy and understanding? How would you describe the practice of medicine?

RESPONDENT: *Frederick Stenn, M.D.*

Physiology has no boundaries, A. J. Carlson used to tell his students. Medicine, too, has no limits. Like the rays of the sun, our art extends its fingers into every phase of human activity. We as practicing physicians learn soon enough that our services are not confined to the pathological and psychiatric understanding of our patient, nor restricted to pill, hypodermic needle, or scalpel. We learn that we have a distinct role as a friend and a counselor, often as a judge, a lawyer, a financier, or an engineer, even as a philosopher, or a minister, mostly as a social worker. We learn that we are treating not disease alone but man too. Ludvig Hektoen exhorted his research workers to "follow through." If a fact is learned, explore it to its greatest depth, he would say. So, too, with the patient, the problem his illness presents to us is merely a small opening which on inquiry leads, like Alice in Wonderland chasing after a rabbit, to a marvelous labyrinth; the deeper we inquire the more effective our therapy.

How frequently we are flattered by the elderly widow smitten by a grave hypertension who asks: "Doctor, shall I sell my home or shall I rent it?"; or the bewildered daughter who asks: "Is it better for me to quit my job and care for my demented mother at home or shall I place her in a sanatorium?"; or the city employee desperately struggling against the effects of a manic-depressive psychosis who earnestly asks: "Is a divorce or a separation the answer to my problem?"; or the parents who grieve over their fifteen-year-old son dying of sarcoma of the spinal cord and who together sit down at our office just to weep and to be reassured; or the young mother with an infant ill with fibrocystic disease of the pancreas who begs: "Doctor, please promise me that my future children will not have this same disease"; or the Bohemian father bowed in sadness who tells again and again the story of the loss of his three sons on the battlefield; or the printer who asks us to appear at the funeral of his seventeen-year-old daughter, dead of myelofibrosis, to give an encouraging word to his heartbroken wife; or the young Greek couple, about to leave for a new home in Alaska who ask: "Doctor, are we doing the right thing?"; or the butcher, pale and thin with cancer that has spread from the larynx to the lumbar spine, who beseeches: "How can I look at death without fear?"; or the Polish wife who says of her husband, home-confined by a stomach tumor: "Doctor, if you'll come around and just talk to him from time to time, he will be able to endure it."

Medicine in its many facets may also include such abilities as: finding a job for a striking steelworker apprehensive over the needs of his four babies; sending a tree to be planted about a home belonging to parents who deserve an appreciative expression for their supreme guidance of their family; writing a note of congratulation on marriage, and a note of consolation at death; calling by phone a dog-kennel operator who is gasping for his breath from congestive heart failure and talking with him about anything but medicine; urging promising girls to take an interest in nursing and teaching as professions; and telegraphing a few roses to a lovely old lady living alone in an attic.

Each day somewhere a doctor grasps the shaking hand of an old man who has just lost his wife and imparts to him the courage necessary to meet the lonely days ahead. Each day somewhere a doctor whispers comforting words into the ears of an expectant woman, exhausted from an arduous and painful labor. Each day somewhere a doctor sits hour after hour at the bedside of his patient critically ill with coronary disease, offering words of cheer and hope. Each day somewhere a doctor gives comfort to the family of the patient who has just undergone a surgical operation. Each day somewhere a doctor sets at ease a mother distressed with the cares of her newborn baby. These and a thousand other similar deeds doctors bring to pass silently and daily all over the world. Indeed, the great leaders of our profession took pride in doing a kindly act, in expressing a gracious thought, in showing that someone cares. Osler, Mackenzie, Broadbent, Parkinson, Lettsom, Shippen, Wistar, Trousseau, Janeway, Da Costa, Weir Mitchell, Dieulafoy, and Diffenback were of this stamp.

Is such magnanimity a part of the function of a doctor? Yes, it is, as much a part as a hammer is the tool of a carpenter. Strict attention to the scientific aspects of a patient is attention to half of a man. Understanding with sympathy, tenderness, and thoughtfulness is the other half. The combination makes a noble medicine.

DIALOGUE OPPORTUNITIES

D. Wayne Montgomery, Th.D.

In 1891, W. L. Schenck was a prophet crying in the wilderness—"The mutual influence of one upon the other [physician and clergyman] would go far towards elevating the race and lessening the tides of disease and misery." [1] Undoubtedly, across the years the listeners have been few. However, there is evidence of the dawning of new efforts. The two professions are drawing nearer with every advance of science.

Dialogue opportunities are twofold. Either they are of a happenstance and oftentimes forced, e.g., the sickroom, or they are designed and structured for a mutual confrontation. The American Medical Association has greatly enhanced the latter through its Committee on Medicine and Religion which has implemented programs on the national, state, and local levels. Personal initiative of those concerned with a total approach to the treatment of man has led to other creative encounters.

Further dialogue and research other than that included in this collection could result in a companion volume treating the personality motive, role analysis, and sharing of knowledge, in the discussion of the meaning of man. It may seem that these are widely divergent topics, but upon closer analysis they are dynamically interrelated.

First of all, the *personality motive* for one's desiring such an interprofessional cooperation must be ascertained. The motive for "engaging" in such a ministry to man cannot casually be laid aside. The ramifications of such a motive could easily affect the resultant relationships between the two professions. A ministerial colleague in a former parish constantly rode on the shirttail of the physicians. His ego building was carried off by constantly alluding in sermon and conversation to "The doctor tells me . . ." It soon became evident to his ministerial colleagues and the physicians of the community that this was no more than an attempt at advertising for counselees—a substitute for "shingle hanging." His personality motive not only alienated him from prospective team members, but also from counselees.

When such an alienation exists there is no chance for dialogue in the clarification of roles, nor is there opportunity for a sharing of knowledge. This type of behavior, among others, is exemplary of that which has made interprofessional cooperation slow in coming.

A physician also needs to identify his reasons for such an engagement. (He can be motivated by personal gain, too!) These do not need to be spelled out, but there is a word of caution to be given here. Religion can become a crutch to compensate for a lazy and inadequate continuing preparation for medical services. While this may draw the pious and nondiscriminating patient to his services, it does little to enhance his position on the healing team.

Second, *role analysis* is essential. If the potential of such a cooperative teamwork in the interest of the whole man is to be realized, then it is imperative that the engaged professions spell out their role expectations and assignments. Each member of the team has to be aware of the clearly defined intricacies to facilitate the execution of his role in the treatment process.

A future volume could beneficially treat the interrelatedness of the two roles. Is it conflictive, compromising, competitive, or complementary? The very fact that the two professions have insights, acquired skills, and knowledge unique to their own profession would make it appear as though they have conflicting goals. Not only do the thought and speech patterns differ, but to one the client is a patient, to the other, a parishioner.

Mendelsohn reports that discussion of the Illinois State Medical Society Committee on Medicine and Religion indicates that a "lack of understanding by the doctor of the clergyman's role

may at times leave the latter feeling that he is forced to function
in an antagonistic environment—and his particular skills are
unwanted, unappreciated and perhaps resented." [2] He further
recognizes that this can be a very real source of frustration in
doctor-clergy relationships.

Role conflict can certainly give rise to role compromise.
There are other factors of compromise to be certain. It is conceivable that the clergyman in his eagerness to be accepted as a
part of the healing team would be reticent or regressive in enacting his assumed role for which he has adequately been trained.

Any minister, who has been at the bedside and engaged in
consultation only to be "interrupted" by the physician, feels the
tendency of compromise as he is in the physician's "domain."
This need not be if the recognition of the role of religion in
patient management was properly understood. A mutual understanding of roles would eliminate the need of compromise on the
part of any participant.

Finally, in regard to role analysis, is it competitive or complementary? The "territorial imperative" principle, the division
of spiritual and physical interests, and nonrecognition of other
professional interests should give way to the newer understanding
of man as a total person. Man viewed in the fourfold aspect of
social, physical, emotional, and spiritual being necessitates both
professions enacting their respective roles in a complementary
manner. It must be realized that their particular skills, insights,
and abilities are not divisive factors, but indeed, are parts of the
whole in an adequate treatment of man. The effective healing
team incorporates both, with each participant realizing the
potential contribution of the other.

With the increased emphasis in theological education on
clinical training, and the proper understanding of his role on the
team, the clergyman can win the respect of the physician and
thereby join together in the treatment of the whole man.

An analysis of the proper relationship of the professions
would include a willingness to *share knowledge*. Much has been
written about the advancements in the preparation of the clergy
to be informed about medical procedures and practices. If cur-

riculum within the two professions is any indication, then the clergy has exceeded the medical profession in learning of the other discipline.

As for the medical profession, it would seem there are two factors to be considered. A doctor should be a student of theology in more than just a layman's interest. Second, he should be willing to accept the clergyman as a tutor in arriving at a more profound understanding of the faith. This is not to deny the fact that some physicians are more accomplished at theology than some ministers! It doesn't take long to detect a physician who is not adept in his field—and, quite conceivably, a physician can detect a minister who has not given himself to the academic pursuit of his tools of trade. By the universal nature of religion it is conceivable that a physician stands the greater chance of exposure to religious knowledge than the clergyman to medical.

Serious questions must be raised concerning the quality of that exposure. There are those theological stances assumed by some medical men which are completely out of keeping with the academic pursuits necessary to be a first-rate physician. It is inconceivable, especially in the light of sociopsychological principles, how a man can cast aside the academic in relation to religion and yet be so reliant upon it for his professional practice. Also, there are instances where the physician lets the dispensing of pills and tracts suffice for a competent practice, which includes an effective interpersonal encounter where the healing process can take place.

A place for alternative tendencies of religious interpretation on the part of the physicians must be recognized. But, when scholarship is overlooked it is inexcusable.

The learning process must be two-way. If man is social, physical, emotional, and spiritual, and if treatment by team effort takes all these factors into consideration, then the physician must be knowledgeable in the area of theology as it is expected the minister should be in medicine. This incorporates a theology of man. The participants in the treatment of the whole man must understand him in dynamic and contextual terms.

Clinebell gives preference to this relationship: "Focusing on

. . . areas of overlapping interest [i.e., the sexual revolution, the terminal patient, euthanasia, ethics of organ transplants, etc.] would seem to be a greater stimulus to interprofessional cooperation than a heavy concentration of the process and problems of this cooperation" (see pages 15–16).

Some participants are capable of moving into a functional relationship at this level. Dialogue of this nature would eventually take into consideration personality motive, role analysis, and sharing of knowledge. That is to say, the newer understandings of man evolving out of dialogue pertaining to the areas of common concern would certainly have implications for other areas of engagement. Wherever the dialogue commences may not be the important factor. What is urgent is that treatment of the whole man cannot be left to a specialist in any one area, but requires the multiple skills and approaches of various disciplines.

Shall we get on with it?

NOTES

The Role of the School and the Community in Sex Education and Related Problems

1. Sidney P. Marland, Jr., "Ferment in the Schools," *Children*, vol. 12 (March–April 1965), p. 65.

2. Leon Eisenberg, "A Developmental Approach to Adolescence," *Children*, vol. 12 (July–August 1965), p. 131.

3. Orville G. Brim, Jr., "Methods of Educating Parents and Their Evaluation," *Prevention of Mental Disorders in Children*, ed. Gerald Caplan (New York: Basic Books, Inc., 1961), p. 133.

4. Thomas E. Shaffer, "Use of Child-Health Conference for Teaching Health and Child Care in High School," *The Journal of School Health*, vol. 19 (1949), p. 155.

5. "School Health Education Study, A Summary Report," *The Study* (Washington, D.C.: 1964).

6. Marian Edgar Breckenridge and E. Lee Vincent, *Child Development* (Philadelphia: W. B. Saunders Co., 1965), p. 405.

7. Sidney Lee Werkman, *The Involvement of Parents in Adolescent Emotional Difficulties in Adolescence, Special Cases and Special Problems* (Washington, D.C.: Catholic University of America Press, 1963).

8. "War on V. D.," *Wall Street Journal* (April 23, 1965).

9. Wayne J. Anderson and Sander M. Latts, "High School Marriages and School Policies in Minnesota," *Journal of Marriage and the Family*, vol. 27 (1965), p. 270.

10. *SIECUS Newsletter* (New York: SIECUS, February 1965).

11. Deryck Calderwood, "Adolescents' Views on Sex Education," *Journal of Marriage and the Family*, vol. 27 (1965), pp. 293–294.

Sex and Mental Health on the Campus

1. Ira L. Reiss, "The Sexual Renaissance: A Summary and Analysis," *The Journal of Social Issues*, vol. 22 (April 1966), pp. 123–137.

2. Alfred Charles Kinsey, et. al., *Sexual Behavior in the Human Female* (Philadelphia: W. B. Saunders Co., 1953).

3. Winston W. Ehrmann, *Premarital Dating Behavior* (New York: Henry Holt & Co., Inc., 1959). See also Mervin B. Freedman, "The Sexual Behavior of American College Women," *Merrill-Palmer Quarterly*, vol. 11 (October 1965), pp. 33–48.

4. Robert E. Grinder and Sue S. Schmitt, "Coeds and Contraceptive In-

formation," *Journal of Marriage and the Family,* vol. 28 (November 1966), p. 471.

5. Harold T. Christensen, "Scandinavian and American Sex Norms: Some Comparisons, with Sociological Implications," *The Journal of Social Issues,* vol. 22 (April 1966), pp. 60–75.

6. Martin B. Loeb, *Social Roles and Sexual Identity in Adolescent Males,* Casework Papers (New York: National Association of Social Workers, 1959).

7. Abraham Harold Maslow, *Motivation and Personality* (New York: Harper & Bros., 1954).

8. Seymour L. Halleck, *Psychiatry and the Dilemmas of Crime* (New York: Harper & Row, Publishers, Inc., 1967).

9. Edmund Bergler, *The Basic Neurosis* (New York: Grune & Stratton, Inc., 1949). See also Margaret Brenman, "On Teasing and Being Teased: and the Problem of 'Moral Masochism,'" *The Psychoanalytic Study of the Child,* vol. 7 (1952), pp. 264–285. Theodor Reik, *Masochism in Modern Man* (New York: Farrar, Straus & Co., 1941).

10. Rollo May, "Antidotes for the New Puritanism," *The Saturday Review,* vol. 49 (March 26, 1966), pp. 19–20.

11. Brenman, *op. cit.*

Extreme Measures to Prolong Life

1. I. M. Rabinowitch, "Euthanasia," *McGill Medical Journal,* vol. 19 (1950), pp. 160–175.

2. E. F. Torrey, "Euthanasia: A Problem in Medical Ethics," *McGill Medical Journal,* vol. 30 (1961), pp. 127–133, 149.

3. Immanuel Jakobovits, "The Dying and Their Treatment in Jewish Law: Preparation for Death and Euthanasia," *Hebrew Medical Journal,* vol. 2 (1961), pp. 245f.

4. Rabinowitch, *op. cit.* See also Torrey, *op. cit.* Joseph Fletcher, "Euthanasia: Our Right to Die," in *Morals and Medicine* (Princeton: Princeton University Press, 1954), pp. 172–210. Willard Learoyd Sperry, *The Ethical Basis of Medical Practice* (New York: Paul B. Hoeber, Inc., 1950), pp. 124–159.

5. Edgar E. Filbey and Kenneth E. Reed, "Some Overtones of Euthanasia," *Hospital Topics,* vol. 43 (September 1965), p. 61.

Prolongation of Life or Prolonging the Act of Dying?

1. Eugene G. Laforet, "The 'Hopeless Case,'" *Archives of Internal Medicine,* vol. 112 (September 1963), p. 317.

2. Edwin J. Holman, "The Law and Artificial Prolongation of Life," read before the Christian Education Committee, United Presbyterian Church, U.S.A. (Chicago, January 12, 1967).

Legal Aspects of the Decision Not to Prolong Life

1. G. L. Williams, "Euthanasia and Abortion," *University of Colorado Law Review,* vol. 38 (1966). See also G. L. Williams, "Mercy-Killing Legislation—A Rejoinder," *Minnesota Law Review,* vol. 43 (1959), p. 1. Y. Kamisar, "Some Non-Religious Views Against Proposed 'Mercy-Killing,' Legislation," *Minnesota Law Review,* vol. 42 (1958), p. 969.

2. Glanville L. Williams, *The Sanctity of Life and the Criminal Law* (New York: Alfred A. Knopf, Inc., 1957). See also Norman St. John-Stevas, *Life, Death and the Law* (London: Eyre & Spottiswoode, 1961).

3. Kamisar, *op. cit.*

4. In 1950, Dr. Herman Sander was brought to trial for injecting air into the veins of one of his cancer-stricken patients. He confessed to the deed, and the attending nurse testified that the patient was still "gasping" when the doctor injected the air. Nonetheless, the motive of mercy prompted the jury of laymen to acquit Dr. Sander (*Time*, Vol. LV [March 6, 1950], p. 20; and *The New York Times* [March 19, 1950], p. 1).

Management of the Patient with Terminal Illness

1. William T. Fitts, Jr., and I. S. Ravdin, "What Philadelphia Physicians Tell Patients With Cancer," *The Journal of the American Medical Association*, vol. 153 (November 7, 1953), pp. 901–904.

2. William B. Bean, "On Death," *Archives of Internal Medicine*, vol. 101 (June 1958), p. 201.

3. Edward V. Stein, "Clergy's Role in Preparing People for and Supporting Them in Catastrophic Illness," read before a workshop of the AMA Committee on Medicine and Religion, San Francisco (June 19, 1964).

4. C. S. Lewis, *The Problem of Pain* (New York: The Macmillan Co., 1962), p. 145.

5. Mark Twain, quoted by Roger J. Bulger, "Doctors and Dying," *Archives of Internal Medicine*, vol. 112 (September 1963), p. 329.

6. Sir Thomas Browne, *The Religio Medici and Other Writings* (London: J. M. Dent & Sons, 1956), p. 43.

7. *Ibid.*, p. 85.

8. Paul Tournier, *Guilt and Grace* (New York: Harper & Brothers, 1962), p. 207.

9. Lewis, *op. cit.*, p. 10.

How Can a Physician Prepare His Patient for Death?

1. Harvey Cushing, *The Life of Sir William Osler*, vol. 2 (Oxford: The Clarendon Press, 1925), p. 620.

2. "Hope," editorial, *Medicine and Science*, vol. 17 (February 1966), p. 90.

3. John S. Stehlin, Jr. and Kenneth H. Beach, "Psychological Aspects of Cancer Therapy," *The Journal of the American Medical Association*, vol. 197 (July 11, 1966), p. 102.

4. Paul S. Rhoads, "Management of the Patient with Terminal Illness," *The Journal of the American Medical Association*, vol. 192 (May 24, 1965), see pp. 149–150 below.

5. Peter F. Regan, "The Dying Patient and His Family," *The Journal of the American Medical Association*, vol. 192 (May 24, 1965), see p. 168 below.

6. Raphael H. Levine, oral communication.

The Dying Patient and His Family

1. Karl Augustus Menninger, *Man Against Himself* (New York: Harcourt Brace, 1938).

2. Alfred Worcester, *Care of Aged, Dying, and the Dead* (Springfield: Charles C. Thomas, 1961).

3. Marc H. Hollender, *Psychology of Medical Practice* (Philadelphia: W. B. Saunders, 1958), pp. 89–115.

4. *Ibid.* See also Donald Oken, "What to Tell Cancer Patients: A Study of Medical Attitudes," *The Journal of the American Medical Association,* vol. 175 (April 1, 1961), pp. 1120–1128.

5. C. Knight Aldrich, "The Dying Patient's Grief," *The Journal of the American Medical Association,* vol. 184 (May 4, 1963), pp. 329–331.

6. Hollender, *op. cit.*

Theories of Ethics and Medical Practice

1. Warner Fite, *Individualism* (New York: Longmans, Green & Co., Inc., 1911).

2. Warner Fite, *The Examined Life* (Bloomington: Indiana University Press, 1957).

3. Paul D. MacLean, "The Limbic System With Respect to Two Basic Life Principles," *The Central Nervous System and Behavior: Transactions of the Second Conference, February 22–25, 1959,* ed. Mary Agnes Burniston Brazier (New York: The Josiah Macy, Jr. Foundation, 1959).

Medical Ethics and Morals in a New Age

1. "Hippocrates, 1966," editorial, *The Journal of the American Medical Association,* vol. 194 (December 20, 1965), pp. 1317–1318.

2. *Percival's Medical Ethics,* ed. C. D. Leake (Baltimore: Williams & Wilkins Co., 1927).

3. American Medical Association, "Principles of Medical Ethics," in *Opinions and Reports of the Judicial Council: Including the Jurisdiction and Rules of the Judicial Council* (Chicago, 1966), p. VI.

4. Robert C. Derbyshire, "What Should the Profession Do About the Incompetent Physician?" *The Journal of the American Medical Association,* vol. 194 (December 20, 1965), p. 1289.

5. Robert E. Hall, "Therapeutic Abortion, Sterilization and Contraception," *American Journal of Obstetrics and Gynecology,* vol. 91 (February 15, 1965), pp. 518–532.

6. "Report of the AMA Board of Trustees Committee on Therapeutic Abortion," in *Proceedings, House of Delegates,* One Hundred and Sixteenth Annual Convention of the American Medical Association (Atlantic City, New Jersey, June 18, 1967), p. 40.

7. "AMA Policy on Therapeutic Abortion," Committee on Human Reproduction, *The Journal of the American Medical Association,* vol. 201 (August 14, 1967), p. 544.

8. George P. Fletcher, "Legal Aspects of the Decision Not to Prolong Life," *The Journal of the American Medical Association,* vol. 203 (January 1, 1968), see p. 141 above.

9. Brian Whitlow, "Extreme Measures to Prolong Life," *The Journal of the American Medical Association,* vol. 202 (October 23, 1967), see p. 126 above.

10. *Ciba Foundation Symposium: Ethics in Medical Progress: With Special Reference to Transplantation,* eds. Gordon Ethelbert Ward Wolstenholme and Maeve O'Connor (Boston: Little, Brown & Co., 1966).

11. *Ibid.,* p. 220.

12. *Ibid.,* p. 75.

13. "Experimentation on Man," editorial, *New England Journal of Medicine,* vol. 274 (June 16, 1966), p. 1383.

14. American Medical Association, *op. cit.,* p. VII.

15. *Sir William Osler: Aphorisms from His Bedside Teachings and Writings,* eds. Robert B. and William B. Bean (Springfield: Charles C. Thomas, Publisher, 1961), p. 91.

16. A. S. Aldis, *Science . . . Its Own Arbiter?* (Lowestoft, East Suffolk: Green & Co.), p. 14.

Dialogue Opportunities

1. W. L. Schenck, "JAMA 75 Years Ago," read before the Forty-Second Annual Meeting of the American Medical Association, Washington, D.C., May 1891, reprinted in *The Journal of the American Medical Association,* vol. 196 (May 23, 1966), p. 20.

2. Robert S. Mendelsohn, "Respect the Clergy, What Every Doctor Should Know About the Religious Needs of His Patients" (Illinois State Medical Society, n.d.), p. 4.

CONTRIBUTORS

Howard J. Clinebell, Jr., Professor of Pastoral Counseling, School of Theology at Claremont, Claremont, California

William Carl Bailey, M.D., Chairman, Denver Medical Society Committee on Medicine and Religion, Denver

Bernard T. Daniels, M.D., Chairman, Colorado Medical Society Committee on Medicine and Religion

Melvin A. Casberg, M.D., Surgeon, Private Practice, Long Beach, California

Alonzo P. Peeke, M.D., Private Practice, Volga, South Dakota

Clarence W. Monroe, M.D., Chief of Plastic Surgery, Children's Memorial Hospital, Chicago

Bob E. Hulit, M.D., Obstetrician and Gynecologist, Private Practice, Billings, Montana

Gotthard Booth, M.D., Psychiatrist, Private Practice, New York City

Abraham N. Franzblau, M.D., Private Practice in Psychoanalytically Oriented Psychotherapy, New York City

Richard P. Bergen, J.D., Director, Legal Research Section, Law Division, American Medical Association, Chicago

Rev. William J. Fogleman, Executive Presbyter, Brazos Presbytery, Presbyterian Church, U.S.

F. P. McKegney, M.D., Associate Professor, Psychiatry and Medicine, Yale University School of Medicine

Julian P. Price, M.D., Head, Department of Pediatrics, The McLeod Infirmary, Florence, South Carolina

Mrs. Malcolm Todd, M.A., Former Principal, Long Beach Retarded Children's Foundation, Long Beach, California

William N. Beachy, M.D., Staff Physician, St. Luke's Hospital, Kansas City, Missouri

E. Mansell Pattison, M.D., Deputy Director, Special Services, County of Orange Community Health Services, Santa Ana, California, and Associate Professor in Residence, Department of Psychiatry and Human Behavior, University of California, Irvine

Paul W. Pruyser, Ph.D., Director, Department of Education, The Menninger Foundation, Topeka, Kansas

William F. Sheeley, M.D., Indiana Mental Health Commissioner, Indianapolis, Indiana

Truman G. Esau, M.D., Psychiatric Consultant, Chicago

Thomas E. Shaffer, M.D., Professor, Department of Pediatrics, Ohio State University, Columbus

Seymour L. Halleck, M.D., Professor of Psychiatry, University of Wisconsin Medical School, Madison

Robert H. Williams, M.D., Professor of Medicine, and Head, Division of Endocrinology, University of Washington, Seattle

Very Rev. Brian Whitlow, D.D., Dean, Anglican Christ Church Cathedral, Victoria, B.C.

Fred Rosner, M.D., Director, Division of Hematology, The Long Island Jewish Hospital, Queens Hospital Center Affiliation, New York

William P. Williamson, M.D., Surgeon, University of Kansas Medical Center, Kansas City, Kansas, deceased

Fred W. Reid, Jr., Chaplain, Assistant Professor of Hospital Administration, University of North Carolina, Chapel Hill

George P. Fletcher, J.D., Assistant Professor of Law, Boston College Law School, Brighton, Massachusetts

Paul S. Rhoads, M.D., Professor Emeritus of Medicine, Northwestern University School of Medicine, Chicago

Willard F. Goff, M.D., Clinical Instructor, Department of Otolaryngology, University of Washington School of Medicine, Seattle

Arthur H. Becker, Ph.D., Professor of Pastoral Care and Social Ethics, Evangelical Lutheran Theological Seminary, Columbus, Ohio

Avery D. Weisman, M.D., Associate Professor of Psychiatry, Massachusetts General Hospital, Harvard Medical School, Boston

Rt. Rev. Msgr. James G. Wilders, Church of St. Thomas More, New York City

Peter F. Regan, M.D., Executive Vice-President, State University of New York, Buffalo

Chauncey D. Leake, Ph.D., Sc.D., Senior Lecturer in Pharmacology and History and Philosophy of Health Professions, School of Medicine, University of California Medical Center, San Francisco, and Past President, The American Medical Association

James Z. Appel, M.D., Private Practice, Lancaster, Pennsylvania

Adolph R. Berger, M.D., Director of Medicine, Goldwater Memorial Hospital, and Professor of Clinical Medicine, New York University Medical Center, New York City

E. G. Shelley, M.D., Private Practice, North East, Pennsylvania

Joseph E. Murray, M.D., Professor of Surgery, Harvard Medical School, Consultant at Peter's and Bent Brigham Children's Hospitals

John L. Lynch, S.J., Professor of Moral Theology, Weston College, Weston, Massachusetts

Kenneth M. Scott, M.D., Director, Christian Medical College and Hospital, Ludhiana, Punjab, India

Robert B. White, M.D., Staff Physician, Health Center, Northern Michigan University, Marquette

Frederick Stenn, M.D., Associate Professor of Medicine, Northwestern University Medical School, Chicago

D. Wayne Montgomery, Th.D., Assistant Professor of Religious Studies, Kansas Wesleyan, Salina, Kansas